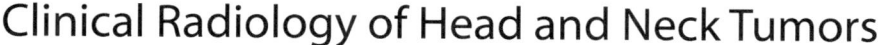

Clinical Radiology of Head and Neck Tumors

Umanath Nayak • Ravikanti Satya Prasad
Shobana Sekhar

Clinical Radiology of Head and Neck Tumors

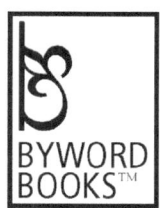

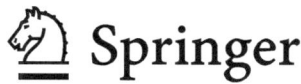

Umanath Nayak
Department of Head and Neck Surgery
and Oncology
Apollo Hospitals
Hyderabad
India

Ravikanti Satya Prasad
Department of Radiology
Apollo Hospitals
Hyderabad
India

Shobana Sekhar
Department of Head and Neck Surgery
and Oncology
Apollo Hospitals
Hyderabad
India

ISBN 978-981-10-5034-3   ISBN 978-981-10-5036-7   (eBook)
https://doi.org/10.1007/978-981-10-5036-7

Library of Congress Control Number: 2017952940

Printed on acid-free paper

Springer Nature Singapore is part of Springer Science+Business Media (www.springer.com)
Byword Books Private Limited, Delhi, India (www.bywordbooks.in)

Foreword

Radiology is an integral part in the management of head and neck tumors. With rapid technological advancements there is a plethora of imaging modalities available to the clinicians. Choosing the best modality for a given clinical situation is of paramount importance to help decide the appropriate treatment. Congratulations to Dr. Nayak, Dr. Prasad, and Dr. Sekhar on bringing out a much needed book on *clinical radiology of head and neck tumors*. This book will be of immense help not only to residents and trainees in the head and neck field but to young consultants as well to help stage, diagnose, and decide on appropriate treatment.

The book is well structured with an initial chapter on normal radiology followed by ten chapters focusing different subsites of the head and neck. Each chapter very lucidly identifies the investigation of choice for the different stages of cancer or particular situations and conditions. It makes easy reading with bullet point presentation and justifications. A number of images of routine clinical scenarios will be an asset to the clinicians when confronted to read an image in the outpatient department. In addition, there are classical images of conditions such as angiofibroma, dumbbell salivary tumor, and paraganglioma where radiology is pathognomonic in establishing the diagnosis. The authors very thoughtfully have listed some of the classical publications in the field at the end for the connoisseurs who desire a more in-depth understanding of the subject.

The book is not a substitute for radiological textbook but is more clinically focused. Two of the authors being surgeons have helped make it more practical and relevant to the clinician. It is a must read for all those concerned with the management of head and neck tumors.

Anil K. Dcruz, MS, DNB, FRCS (Hon)
Chief of Head and Neck Services and Director
Tata Memorial Hospital
Mumbai, India

Preface

This book is a quick reference guide to the busy clinician in understanding the radiology of head and neck tumors in a simple and lucid manner.

Imaging plays a vital role in the better understanding and management of any pathology in the human body and head and neck tumors are no different. With the wide range of imaging modalities currently available and frequent upgrades in technology and image resolution, the clinician is often in a dilemma as to which modality would be best suited for a certain condition. Balancing the advantages of the investigation ordered and the clinician's familiarity with that imaging modality with the costs incurred and patient inconveniences/risks can sometimes be a daunting task, and it is our endeavor with this book to help the clinician come to a decision in the form of case studies described. This book does not attempt to address all aspects of head and neck radiology but addresses imaging options for head and neck tumors alone. The primary focus is on the two frequently used modalities of imaging for head and neck tumors—CT and MR—and while a mention is made of the other modalities and their role wherever applicable, the reader is advised to refer to the reading list at the end of the chapter for further information.

The book is presented in the form of pictorial illustrations based on the clinical conditions patients present with as we believe that this may be the best way for the clinician to understand the radiology of that disease. Wherever possible an attempt has been made to show the CT and MR images of the same condition side-by-side for comparison. Normal radiology is presented as a separate chapter at the beginning of the book, and the reader is advised to first familiarize himself/herself with the normal images described in this chapter and refer to it when needed for a better understanding of the pathologic processes in the later chapters.

Often the clinician has access to only limited images available in the radiology films handed over to the patient—CDs sometimes provided contain more images, but the process of opening them can sometimes be time-consuming and most clinicians are not particularly fond of going through that extra trouble. On the other hand, the radiologist has the advantage of access to the entire sequence of images saved as well as the option of reconstructing these images in coronal, sagittal sequence etc., and it is therefore important that the clinician communicate with the radiologist when in doubt for further clarity. Often a quick visit to the radiology unit and studying the entire sequence of images in the monitors can be extremely informative.

We sincerely hope that the book will help in the better understanding of imaging of head and neck tumors.

Hyderabad, India   Umanath Nayak
Hyderabad, India   Ravikanti Satya Prasad
Hyderabad, India   Shobana Sekhar

Contents

About the Authors

Umanath Nayak is the chief and senior consultant at the Department of Head and Neck Surgery at the Apollo Hospitals, Hyderabad, India, and director of the Fellowship Program. He is a fellow of the University of California, Davis, and was twice awarded UICC fellowships for projects in London and Amsterdam. He is the editor of the book *Voice Restoration After Total Laryngectomy* and two other books related to cancer. (e-mail: drumanathnayak@gmail.com)

Ravikanti Satya Prasad is a senior consultant radiologist at the Department of Radiology and Imaging Sciences at the Apollo Hospitals, Hyderabad, and director of the Academic Program. He was previously the chief of radiology at Lanka Hospitals, Colombo, Sri Lanka. (e-mail: drprasad4893@gmail.com)

Shobana Sekhar is a junior consultant at the Department of Head and Neck Surgery at the Apollo Hospitals, Hyderabad. She has a masters in Oral and Maxillofacial Surgery and a Fellowship in Head and Neck Oncology and has trained in microvascular free flap surgery. (e-mail: shobanasekhar@gmail.com)

Normal Imaging

This chapter focuses on the role of different imaging modalities in the evaluation of head and neck tumors and in understanding and comparing normal CT and MR at different levels in the head and neck.

Choice of Imaging

1. **Computed tomography (CT) with contrast**
   (a) It is the most common and popular modality for imaging head and neck tumors in view of clinician familiarity and patient convenience.
   (b) It is fast, well tolerated, and readily available but has lower contrast resolution when compared to MR and requires iodinated contrast and ionizing radiation. It is less expensive compared to MR.
   (c) It is the best modality for assessing bony and vascular structures and their involvement.
   (d) CT is superior to other imaging modalities for assessing lung and bone secondaries in H & N cancer.
   (e) Contrast enhanced CT (CECT) is the preferred imaging modality for assessing head and neck tumors. Most tumors pick up contrast well, and this helps delineate it from the surrounding soft tissues. However, a baseline non-contrast (Plain) study should necessarily precede the contrast study.
   (f) While plain CT by itself has a limited role in the assessment of head and neck tumors and is generally reserved for trauma and infection, it is a necessary part of the evaluation process and should be done before administering the contrast. Though it may add to the dose of radiation that the patient is exposed to, plain CT can serve as a baseline study to compare the degree and pattern of the enhancement as well as to identify certain things such as calcifications and hemorrhage into a tumor which may be missed on contrast CT.

© The Author(s) 2018
U. Nayak et al., *Clinical Radiology of Head and Neck Tumors*,
https://doi.org/10.1007/978-981-10-5036-7_1

(g) The use of bone and soft tissue windows (which can be adjusted manually using computer settings) can further aid in better visualization of the structures of interest.

(h) While axial CT continues to be the default image acquisition, sagittal and coronal reconstruction has greatly added to the overall understanding of the disease process and its extensions.

(i) It is important to keep in mind that radiation exposure from CT is much higher compared to other modalities and therefore CT at frequent intervals must be avoided wherever possible. An average CT of the neck with contrast exposes one to about 7–15 mSv (millisievert) of radiation—equivalent to radiation exposure from approx 100–150 chest radiographs (one chest X-ray exposes a person to 0.1 mSv of radiation). CT scans are contraindicated during pregnancy due to the risks to the fetus.

(j) Iodinated contrast is used for contrast enhanced CT. Since it is nephrotoxic, a serum creatinine is recommended as a routine before performing the study. Patients with CKD may have deterioration of their renal function following administration of the contrast, and the advantages of the use of this modality should be balanced against the risks of renal failure. It is advised to take a nephrologist's opinion prior to undertaking the study. The use of contrast is also contraindicated in patients with known sensitivity to iodine.

(k) Head and neck CT imaging is generally performed from the level of the clivus to the aortic arch. Two millimeter slices are preferred. The currently popular CT machine is 64-slice and allows fast imaging, excellent resolution, and good reconstruction in both coronal and sagittal planes.

   Note: Unless otherwise specified, all CT images in this book are contrast enhanced CTs (CECTs).

2. **Magnetic resonance imaging (MRI)**

(a) Though traditionally used in the head and neck for problem-solving when CT findings are equivocal, MR is gradually gaining popularity for primary assessment of head and neck tumors.

(b) MRI has the advantages of higher soft tissue contrast resolution, the lack of iodine-based contrast agents, and high sensitivity for perineural and intracranial disease.

(c) The disadvantages of MRI include lower patient tolerance, contraindicated in patients with pacemakers and certain other implanted metallic devices, and artifacts related to multiple causes, not the least of which is motion.

(d) Although inferior compared to CT in assessing bone erosion, early marrow invasion is better demonstrated on MR than CT.

(e) It is the imaging modality of choice for head and neck tumors with intracranial spread. Dura, brain and cavernous sinus invasion, perineural spread, and orbital extensions are very well demonstrated by MR. It is also the modality of choice for the evaluation of CSF rhinorrhea/otorrhea.

(f) The availability of different sequences (T1 with or without contrast, T2, STIR, DWI, etc.) *(refer TABLE 1.1 below)* is an added advantage with this

Table 1.1 Tissue characteristics for CT and various MR sequences

	Plain CT	Contrast CT	MR T1	MR T2	Contrast MR	MR STIR (fat suppressed)
BONE	Bright	Bright	Dark	Dark	Dark	Dark
FAT	Dark	Dark	Bright	Bright	Bright	Dark
FLUID	Dark	Dark	Dark	Bright	Dark	Bright
MUSCLE	Dark	Dark (mild enhancement compared to plain)	Intermediate	Intermediate	Uniform enhancement	Same as T2 (interfasicular fat suppressed)
BLOOD VESSELS	Dark	Bright	Dark (flow void)	Dark	Bright	Bright
TUMOR	Dark	Bright	Dark (except in fat containing tumors)	Bright	Bright	Depending on fat
LYMPHNODE	Hypodense	Bright	Intermediate with central bright hilar fat	Intermediate	Bright	Intermediate with suppressed hilar fat
LIGAMENTS	Dark	Dark	Dark	Dark	Dark	Dark
NERVE	Hypodense	Hypodense	Intermediate	Intermediate	Intermediate	Intermediate
AIR-FILLED SPACES	Dark	Dark	Dark	Dark	Dark	Dark

modality. The equipment also allows images to be taken in all three views (axial, coronal, sagittal) unlike with CT where coronal and sagittal have to be reconstructed from axial images.

(g) The prolonged time taken for imaging and requirement for patient to lay still in a closed chamber can be difficult for children, older patients as well as those that are sick and claustrophobic.

(h) Since there is no radiation exposure from an MR study, its use is safe in pregnancy (though use of contrast is contraindicated in pregnancy).

(i) Gadolinium is used as contrast for MR. Being non-iodinated, it can be safely used in patients sensitive to iodine. Patients with CKD (Stage 3 and above) are advised against use of Gadolinium due to possibility of development of nephrogenic systemic fibrosis (NSF). Fortunately, since MR has many imaging sequences (DWI, STIR, FAT SUPPRESSED, etc.) one may still do imaging in CKD patients avoiding contrast.

   (j) Since a powerful magnet is one of the components of the equipment used for
       the study, metallic implants, pacemaker, etc. are at risk of dislodgement/
       malfunction and use of this modality in patients possessing these is rela-
       tively contraindicated and needs to be done with care.
   (k) The unit Tesla determines the magnetic strength of an MR machine. Ideally,
       1.5 T and above is recommended as DWI is only possible with this. The
       higher the Tesla better is the resolution and faster is the imaging.
3. **Ultrasonography (USG)**
   (a) Simplicity, ease of performance, and low cost make it a preferred modality
       for initial evaluation of neck masses and subclinical neck secondaries.
   (b) It is the primary modality in evaluation of thyroid nodules and parathyroid
       disease and can also assist in guided biopsies (FNAC and Tru-cut) of head
       and neck tumors.
   (c) It is a real-time study.
   (d) Addition of color Doppler adds advantages in terms of assessment of
       vascularity of the lesions and the surroundings and helps avoid vascular
       structures during guided biopsies.
   (e) Although easily available and free of any radiation exposure, it is dependent
       on the experience and subjectivity of the performing radiologist and images
       may not allow for easy comprehension by the clinician.
4. **Positron emission tomography (PET) CT**
   (a) It is a modality which combines PET scan with CT images and gives an
       amalgation of biological imaging (PET) with anatomical imaging (CT).
       Malignant tumors show higher glucose uptake, and this property is utilized
       to identify pathological lesions.
   (b) It is the imaging modality of choice for post-RT/post-surgical relapses as it
       can consistently differentiate edema and fibrosis from tumor.
   (c) In lymphomas, it is valuable in the initial staging as well as in assessment of
       treatment response and follow-up.
   (d) Though the PET component has limited radiation exposure, the CT compo-
       nent exposes patient to a high radiation dose.
   (e) It is necessary to monitor patient's blood sugar levels before doing the
       study as the radio-pharmaceutical used for the study is glucose based
       (Fluorodeoxyglucose—FDG)
   (f) The disadvantages are its limited availability, high cost and the fact that
       inflammatory lesions may also demonstrate higher uptake and result in false
       positives.
5. **Plain radiographs**
   (a) Plain radiography has a limited role in the evaluation of head and neck
       lesions; however, neck radiographs can show hypertrophied adenoids, for-
       eign bodies in aerodigestive tract, position of the trachea, cervical spine
       alignment, vertebral erosions and destruction.

(b) Chest X-ray: It is used in the routine evaluation of patients with head and neck cancer. It aids in assessing pulmonary status, position and compression of trachea in large thyroid masses, and the presence of possible lung metastasis.

(c) Orthopantamogram of the mandible (OPG): A simple and inexpensive modality to assess involvement of mandible in oral cavity lesions.

6. **Technetium thyroid scan**

   Commonly done in the assessment of hyperthyroid status to differentiate between Graves' disease, toxic nodules, and secondary hyperthyroidism.

7. **Radioiodine scan**

   Used in the postsurgical evaluation of residual thyroid and metastatic disease in Ca thyroid as well as in follow-up of high risk patients after treatment.

8. **Miscellaneous**

   Other uncommonly used modalities in the head and neck are SPECT scan for parathyroid localization, assessment of cerebral perfusion, and for localizing metastasis in thyroid cancers; DEXA scan for evaluation of bone density, Gadolinium scan for tumors secreting catecholamine, Tc Sestamibi scan for evaluation of hyperparathyroidism.

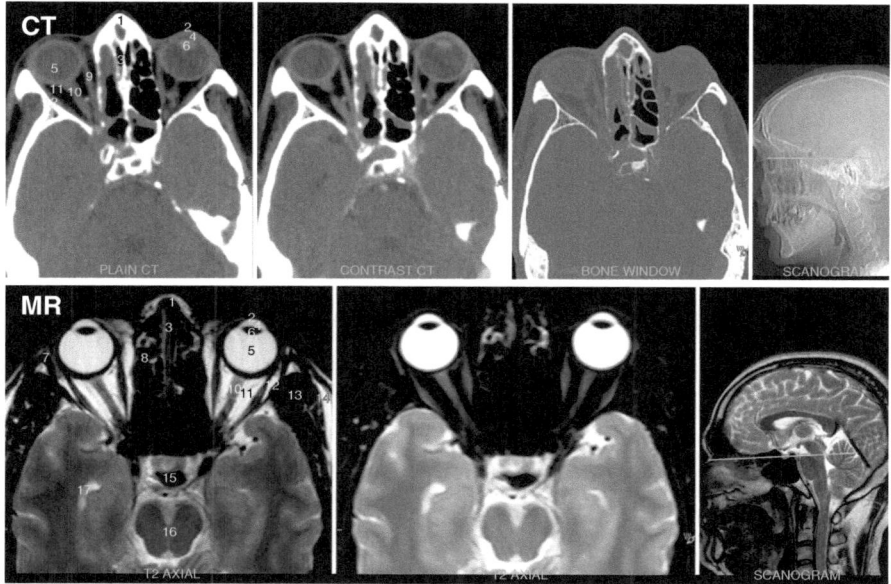

Fig. 1.1 Orbit. (*1*) Nasal bone, (*2*) Cornea, (*3*) Nasal septum, (*4*) Anterior chamber, (*5*) Eyeball, (*6*) Lens, (*7*) Zygomatic bone, (*8*) Ethmoid air cells, (*9*) Medial rectus, (*10*) Optic nerve, (*11*) Retro-orbital fatty tissue, (*12*) Lateral rectus, (*13*) Sphenoid bone, (*14*) Temporalis muscle, (*15*) Pituitary gland, (*16*) Mid brain, (*17*) Temporal horn of lateral ventricle

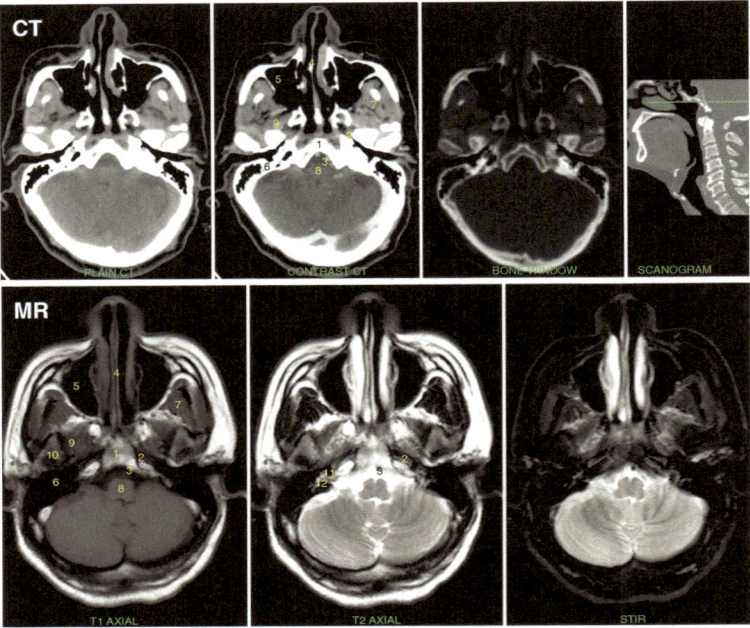

Fig. 1.2 Clivus. (*1*) Clivus, (*2*) Internal carotid artery (ICA), (*3*) Basilar artery, (*4*) Nasal septum, (*5*) Maxillary sinus, (*6*) Petrous bone, (*7*) Infratemporal fossa, (*8*) Medulla, (*9*) Lateral pterygoid muscle, (*10*) Mandibular condyle, (*11*) Cochlea, (*12*) Vestibule

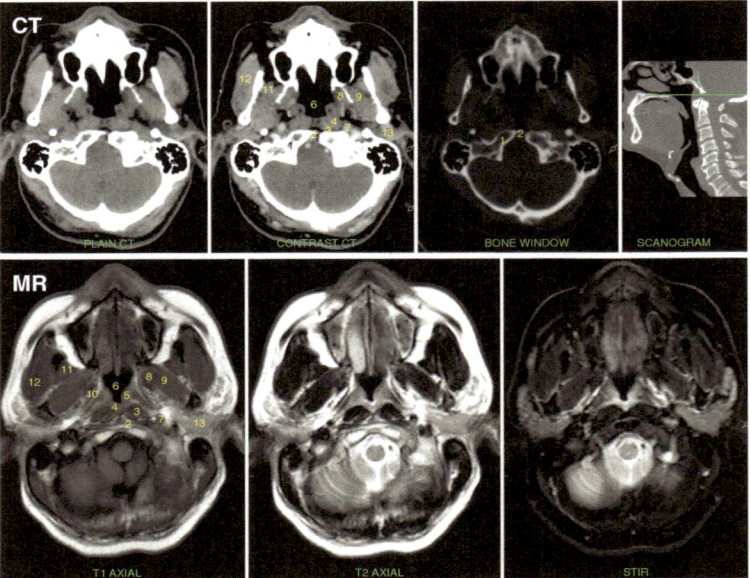

Fig. 1.3 Occipital condyle. (*1*) Occipital condyle, (*2*) Anterior arch of atlas, (*3*) Longus capitis, (*4*) Splenius capitis, (*5*) Levator veli palatini, (*6*) Nasopharynx, (*7*) ICA, (*8*) Medial pterygoid, (*9*) Lateral pterygoid, (*10*) Tensor veli palatini, (*11*) Temporalis, (*12*) Masseter, (*13*) Parotid gland

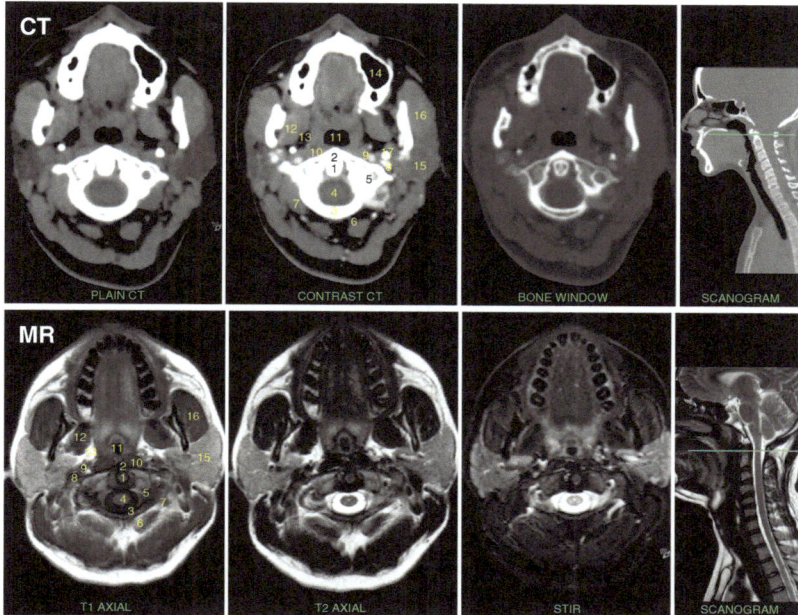

Fig. 1.4 Atlanto-axial joint. (*1*) Odontoid process, (*2*) Anterior arch of atlas, (*3*) Posterior arch of atlas, (*4*) Spinal cord, (*5*) Vertebral artery, (*6*) Rectus capitis, (*7*) Rectus capitis lateralis, (*8*) IJV, (*9*) ICA, (*10*) Longus capitis, (*11*) Pharynx, (*12*) Pterygoid muscles, (*13*) Parapharyngeal space, (*14*) Maxillary sinus, (*15*) Parotid, (*16*) Masseter, (*17*) Styloid process

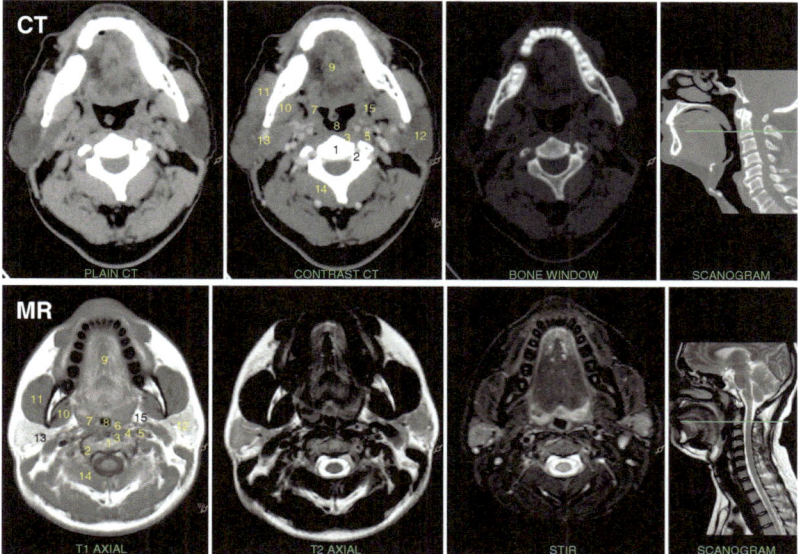

Fig. 1.5 C2 body. (*1*) Body of C2, (*2*) Vertebral artery, (*3*) Longus Colli, (*4*) Longus capitis, (*5*) ICA, (*6*) Superior constrictor, (*7*) Palato-pharyngeus, (*8*) Oropharynx, (*9*) Genioglossus, (*10*) Medial pterygoid, (*11*) Masseter, (*12*) Parotid gland, (*13*) Retromandibular vein, (*14*) Splenius capitis, (*15*) Parapharyngeal space

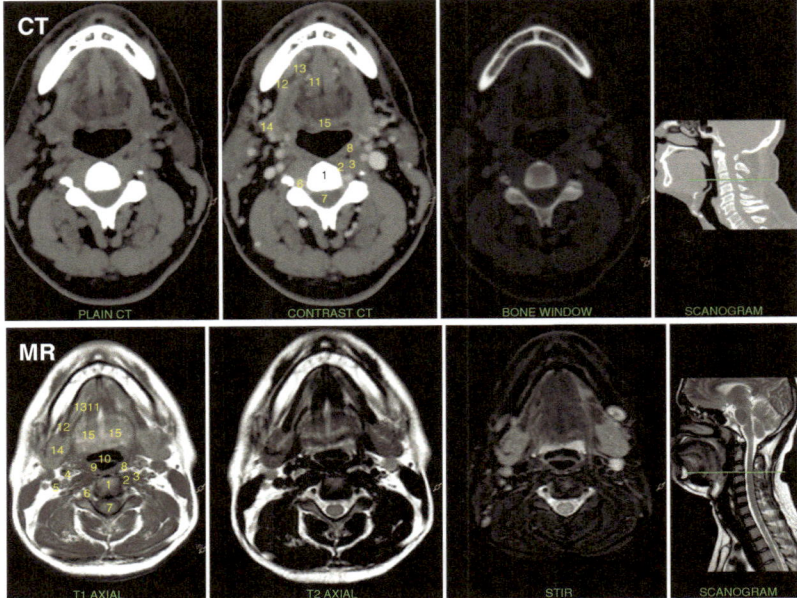

Fig. 1.6 C3 body. (*1*) C3 body, (*2*) Longus colli, (*3*) Longus capitis, (*4*) External carotid artery (ECA), (*5*) ICA, (*6*) Vertebral artery, (*7*) Spinal cord, (*8*) Middle constrictor, (*9*) Palatoglossus, (*10*) Epiglottis, (*11*) Genioglossus, (*12*) Mylohyoid, (*13*) Hyoglossus, (*14*) Submandibular gland, (*15*) Base of tongue

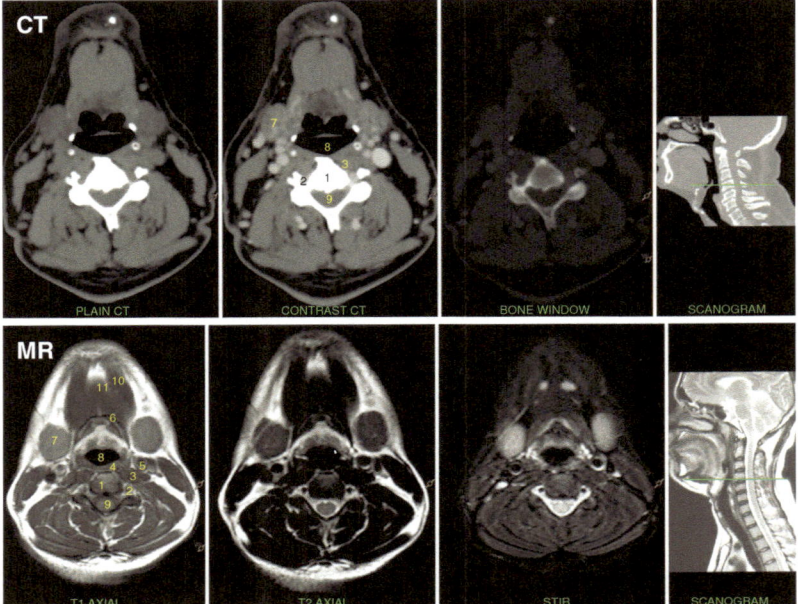

Fig. 1.7 C4 body. (*1*) C4 body, (*2*) Vertebral artery, (*3*) Longus Colli, (*4*) Inferior constrictor muscles, (*5*) Common carotid artery, (*6*) Hyoid bone, (*7*) Submandibular gland, (*8*) Laryngeal vestibule, (*9*) Spinal cord, (*10*) Anterior belly of digastric muscle, (*11*) Mylohyoid

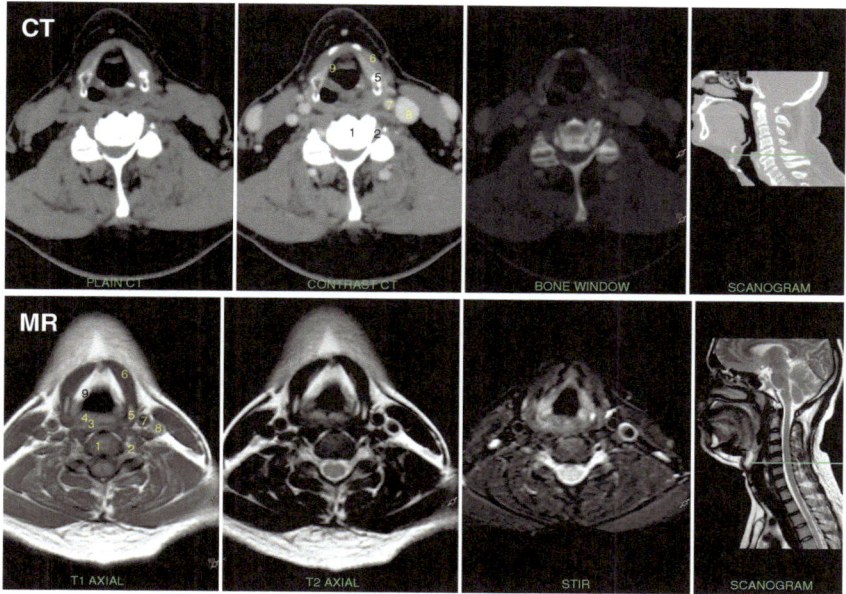

Fig. 1.8 C5 body. (*1*) C5 body, (*2*) Vertebral artery, (*3*) Inferior constrictor, (*4*) Posterior Crico-arytenoid muscle, (*5*) Thyroid cartilage, (*6*) Strap muscles, (*7*) Common carotid artery, (*8*) Internal jugular vein, (*9*) False cords

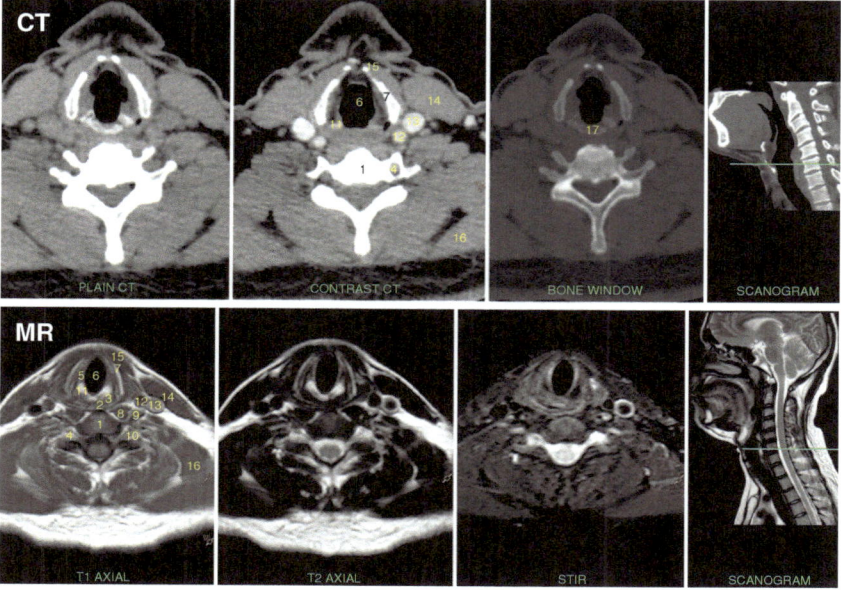

Fig. 1.9 C6 body. (*1*) C6 body, (*2*) Inferior constrictor, (*3*) Posterior crico-arytenoid muscle, (*4*) Vertebral artery, (*5*) Vocalis muscle, (*6*) Glottis opening, (*7*) Thyroid cartilage, (*8*) Longus colli, (*9*) Longus capitis, (*10*) Spinal nerve root, (*11*) Arytenoid cartilage, (*12*) CCA, (*13*) Internal Jugular vein, (*14*) Sternocleidomastoid muscle, (*15*) Strap muscles, (*16*) Trapezius muscle, (*17*) Posterior arch of cricoid (CT—bone window)

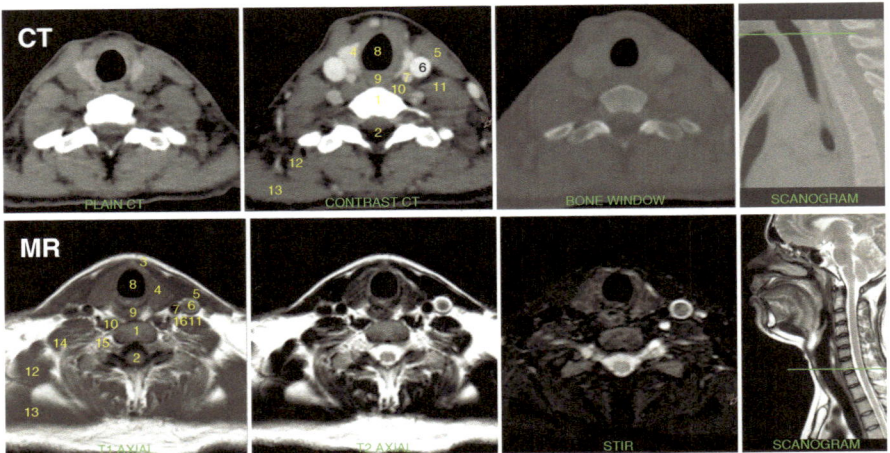

Fig. 1.10 C7 body. (*1*) C7 Vertebra, (*2*) Spinal Cord, (*3*) Sternohyoid muscle, (*4*) Thyroid gland, (*5*) Sternocleidomastoid muscle, (*6*) IJV, (*7*) CCA, (*8*) Trachea, (*9*) Oesophagus, (*10*) Longus colli, (*11*) Anterior scalene muscle, (*12*) Levator scapule, (*13*) Trapezius, (*14*) Posterior scalene muscle, (*15*) Vertebral artery, (*16*) Vagus

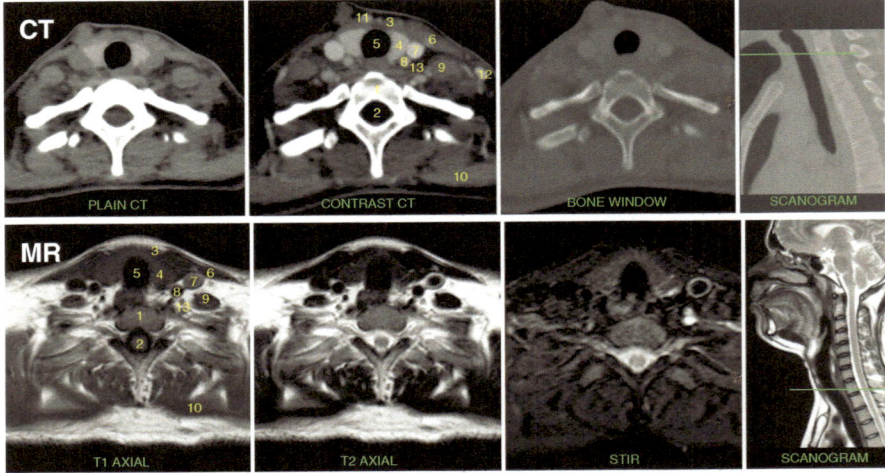

Fig. 1.11 D1 body. (*1*) Body of T1, (*2*) Spinal cord, (*3*) Sternohyoid, (*4*) Thyroid, (*5*) Trachea, (*6*) Sternocleidomastoid, (*7*) IJV, (*8*) Common carotid artery, (*9*) Anterior scalene muscle, (*10*) Trapezius, (*11*) Anterior jugular vein, (*12*) External jugular vein, (*13*) Vagus

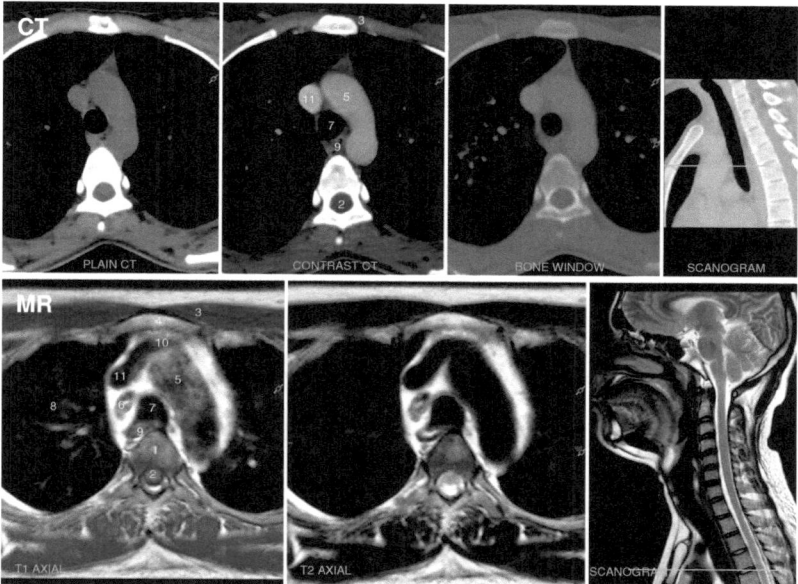

Fig. 1.12 Aortic arch (D4). (*1*) T4 Vertebra, (*2*) Spinal cord, (*3*) Pectoralis major muscle, (*4*) Sternum, (*5*) Arch of aorta, (*6*) Paratracheal Lymph node, (*7*) Trachea, (*8*) Lung, (*9*) Oesophagus, (*10*) Left brachiocephalic vein, (*11*) Superior vena cava

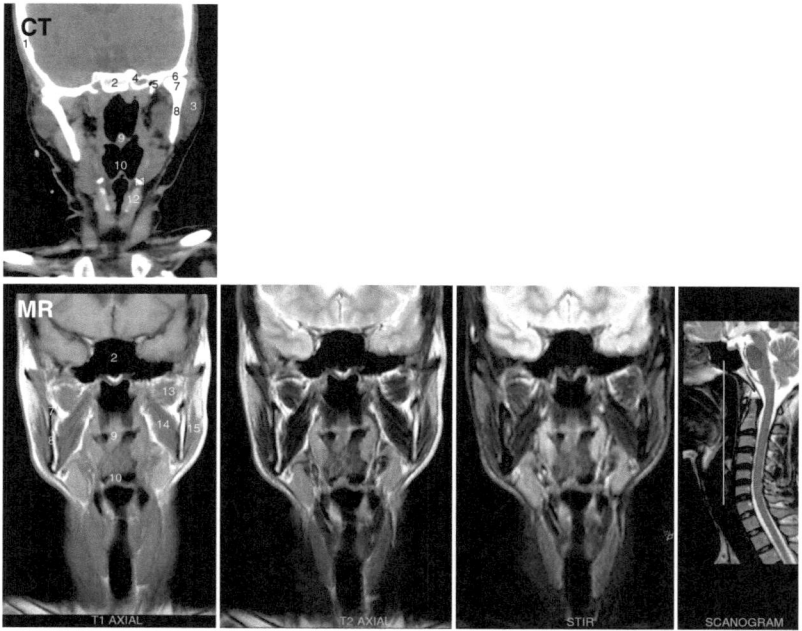

Fig. 1.13 Upper aero-digestive tract—coronal. (*1*) Frontal bone, (*2*) Body of sphenoid bone, (*3*) Parotid gland, (*4*) Petrous part of temporal bone, (*5*) Spine of sphenoid bone, (*6*) Temporomandibular joint, (*7*) Head of mandible, (*8*) Ramus of mandible, (*9*) Uvula, (*10*) Epiglottis, (*11*) Hyoid bone, (*12*) Thyroid cartilage, (*13*) Lateral Pterygoid, (*14*) Medial Pterygoid, (*15*) Masseter

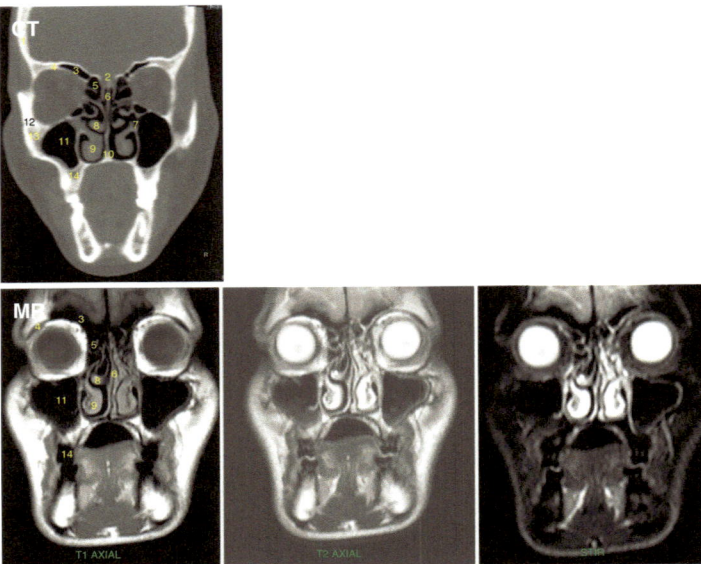

Fig. 1.14 PNS—coronal. (*1*) Frontal bone, (*2*) Crista galli, (*3*) Frontal sinus, (*4*) Roof of orbit, (*5*) Ethmoid air cells, (*6*) Nasal septum, (*7*) Uncinate process, (*8*) Middle turbinate, (*9*) Inferior turbinate, (*10*) Vomer, (*11*) Maxillary sinus, (*12*) Frontozygomatic suture, (*13*) Zygomatic bone, (*14*) Maxillary bone

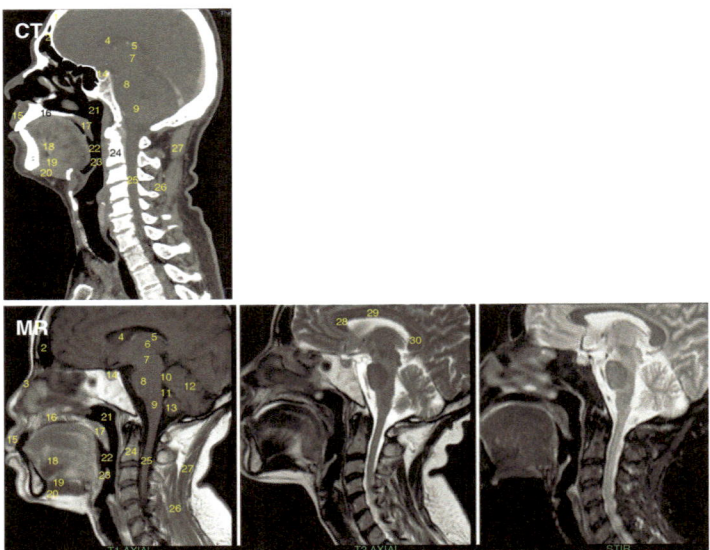

Fig. 1.15 Mid-sagittal. (*1*) Frontal bone, (*2*) Frontal sinus, (*3*) Nasal bone, (*4*) Lateral ventricle, (*5*) Internal cerebral vein, (*6*) Thalamus, (*7*) Mid brain, (*8*) Pons, (*9*) Medulla, (*10*) Superior cerebellar peduncle, (*11*) Fourth ventricle, (*12*) Cerebellum, (*13*) Cerebellar tonsil, (*14*) Pituitary gland, (*15*) Orbicularis oris, (*16*) Hard palate, (*17*) Soft palate, (*18*) Genioglossus, (*19*) Geniohyoid, (*20*) Mylohyoid, (*21*) Nasopharynx, (*22*) Oropharynx, (*23*) Epiglottis, (*24*) Axis vertebra, (*25*) Spinal cord, (*26*) Splenius capitis, (*27*) Trapezius, (*28*) Corpus callosum genu, (*29*) Corpus callosum body, (*30*) Corpus callosum splenium

Choice of Imaging

1. **OPG (orthopantomogram)** is a relatively simple and inexpensive plain radiograph that can provide useful preliminary information regarding mandible involvement and dental status.
2. **CT** is the primary modality of imaging in oral cancer and can provide detailed information about the extent of bone involvement (mandible and maxillary alveolus/hard palate), paramandibular disease, extension into infratemporal fossa/pterygoid muscle invasion—information that can impact on patient management.
3. **MR** is of great value in assessing deep invasion in case of deeply infiltrating tongue and floor of mouth cancer and thus determine approach (intraoral approach/mandibulotomy) as well as early invasion of mandibular marrow where CT findings may be equivocal.
4. Both CT and MR (as well as ultrasound in experienced hands) can give a high degree of accuracy in identifying subclinical lymph node involvement in N0 neck and assist the clinician in the decision whether to perform elective neck dissection or not (in early cancers).
5. **PET-CT** is the imaging of choice to assess postsurgical/post-CTRT relapse to differentiate recurrence from fibrosis and postsurgical changes.

Early Disease (T1T2)

1. Imaging in early oral cancer (usually CT) is utilized for assessing early cortical invasion in tumors adjacent to bone (mandible in case of disease involving lower gingivum/GB sulcus and maxillary alveolus/hard palate in case of upper gingivum/GB sulcus).
2. In retromolar trigone lesion, both CT and MR can give good information about involvement of IT (infratemporal) fossa.

© The Author(s) 2018
U. Nayak et al., *Clinical Radiology of Head and Neck Tumors*,
https://doi.org/10.1007/978-981-10-5036-7_2

3. A routine CT/MR in situations other than those mentioned above may not usually provide any further clinically relevant information about the primary disease beyond what can be obtained from a thorough clinical examination.

4. USG neck is often of help in assessing neck node status in doubtful cases and may aid in the decision to perform an elective neck dissection. It can also serve as a baseline for further follow-up of the neck in cases which are kept on neck observation.

5. A puffed cheek maneuver is often employed to diagnose early gingivo-buccal cancers and their local extensions.

Advanced Disease (T3T4)

1. Imaging is vital in all cases of advanced oral cancer and can provide valuable additional information beyond clinical examination, e.g., extent and degree of bone involvement, soft tissue extension of disease, infratemporal/skull base extension, proximity to carotid artery, deep (extrinsic muscle) involvement in case of Ca tongue.

2. CT/MR will also be able to differentiate operable from inoperable disease.

Fig. 2.1 (a) OPG mandible showing unilocular cyst suggestive of benign odontogenic cyst. (b) OPG mandible showing gross involvement by Gingivo-buccal cancer

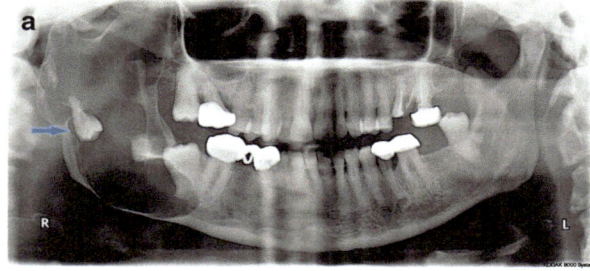

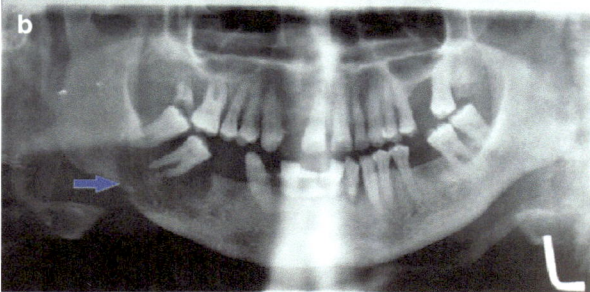

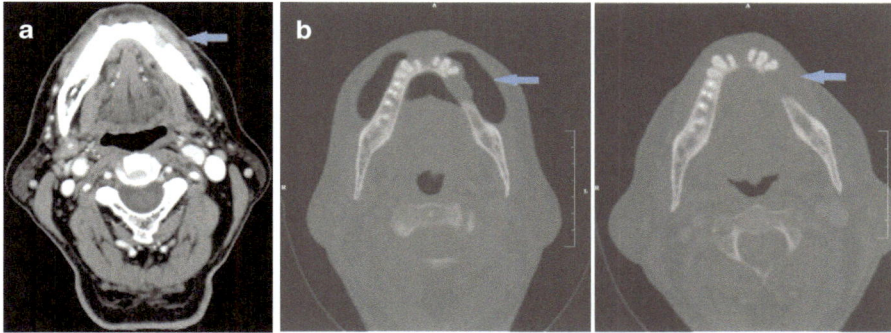

Fig. 2.2 (a) Ca lower alveolus. Axial CT (soft tissue window) showing early cortical destruction. Stage T2—amenable to marginal mandibulectomy. (b) Ca lower alveolus same patient (bone windows). Puffed cheek manoeuvre showing tumor in picture on left

Fig. 2.3 (**a**) Ca upper GB sulcus with erosion of upper alveolus—axial CT. (**b**) Ca upper GB sulcus (same patient) Coronal reconstruction

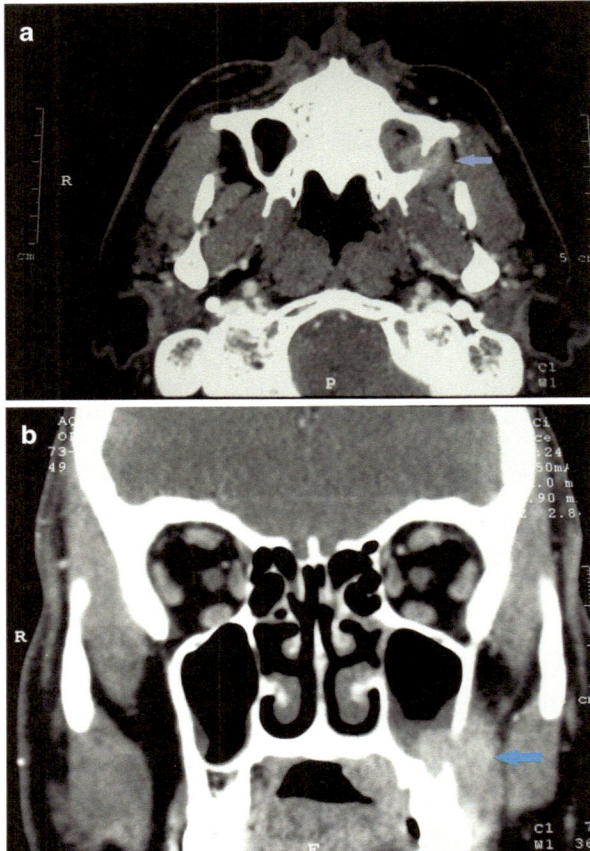

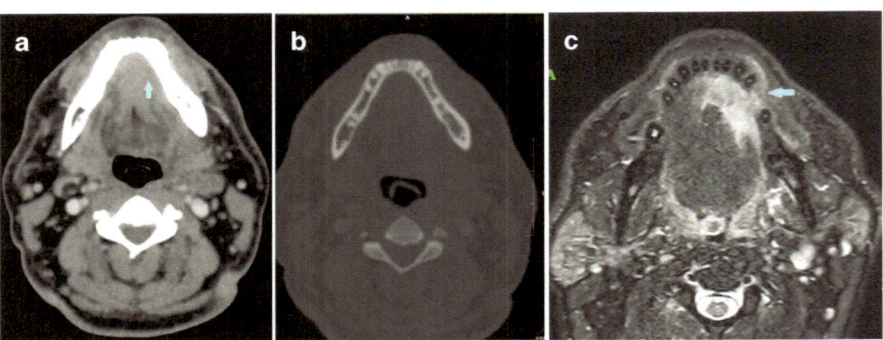

Fig. 2.4 Ca Floor of mouth (**a**) Contrast CT showing lesion floor of mouth abutting lingual cortex mandible – mandible does not show any involvement Stage T3 (**b**) Bone window showing no obvious bone involvement (**c**) T2 axial MRI of same patient showing early marrow invasion (missed on CT) along with the lesion in floor of mouth – upstaged to T4

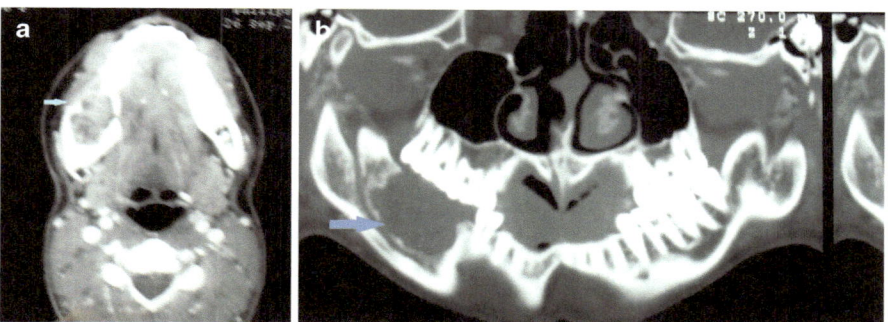

Fig. 2.5 (**a**) Ameloblastoma with bi-cortical expansion of mandible. (**b**) Ameloblastoma mandible—CT OPG—may be used to get an accurate idea of the extent of bone excision and subsequent reconstruction

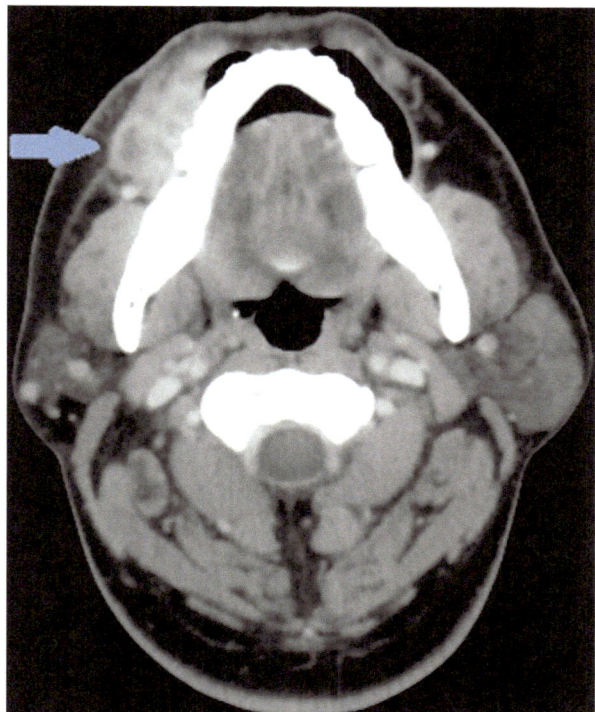

Fig. 2.6 Ca buccal mucosa with paramandibular disease, no bone erosion

Fig. 2.7 Ca buccal
mucosa Coronal CT
demonstrating
paramandibular disease.
Note tumor extension to
upper GB sulcus

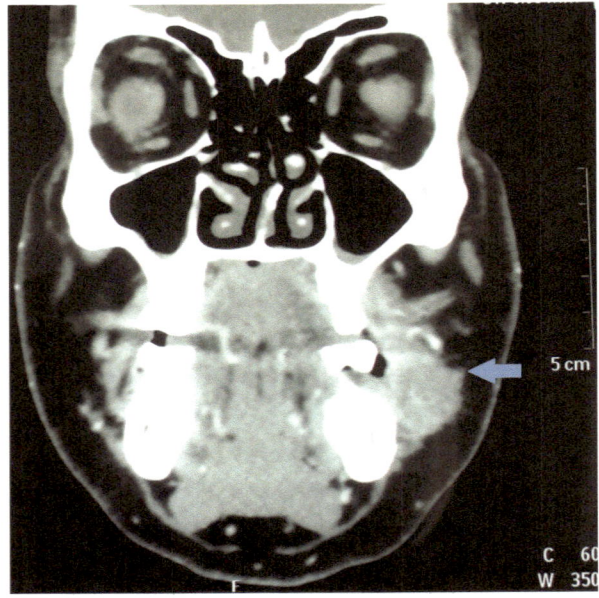

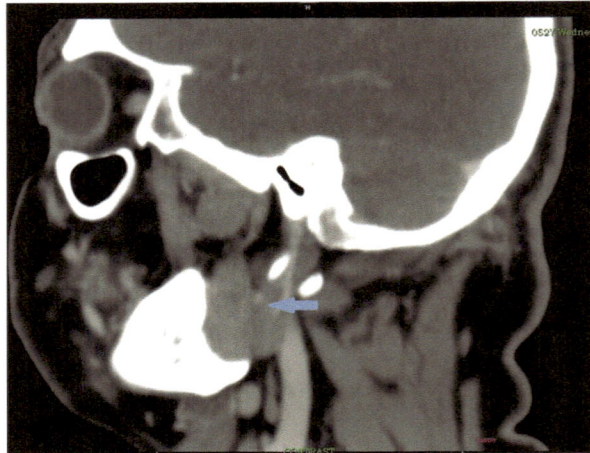

Fig. 2.8 Ca buccal mucosa
Sagittal CT to demonstrate
paramandibular disease.
Though there is no
mandible involvement
patient will require
segmental resection of
mandible

Fig. 2.9 Advanced oral Ca with gross mandibular invasion (T4). Note involvement of tongue and pharyngo-mucosal space and necrotic Level II node

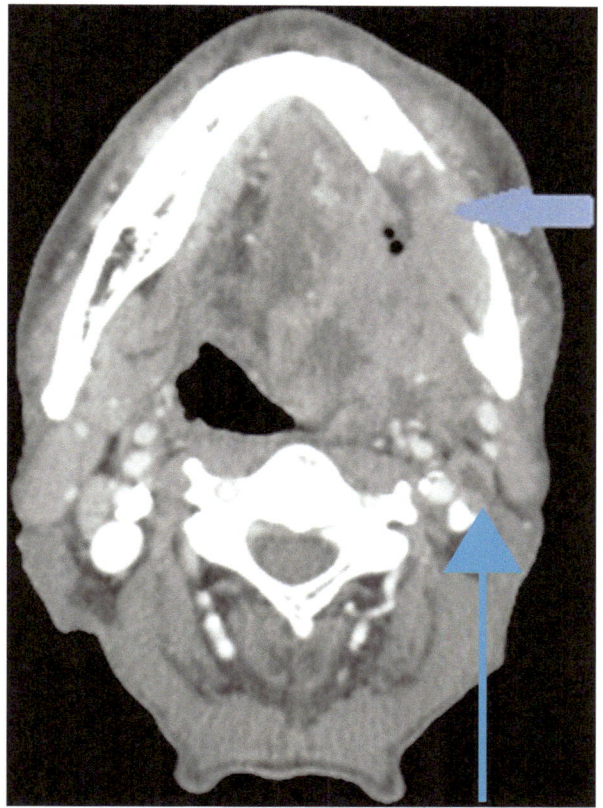

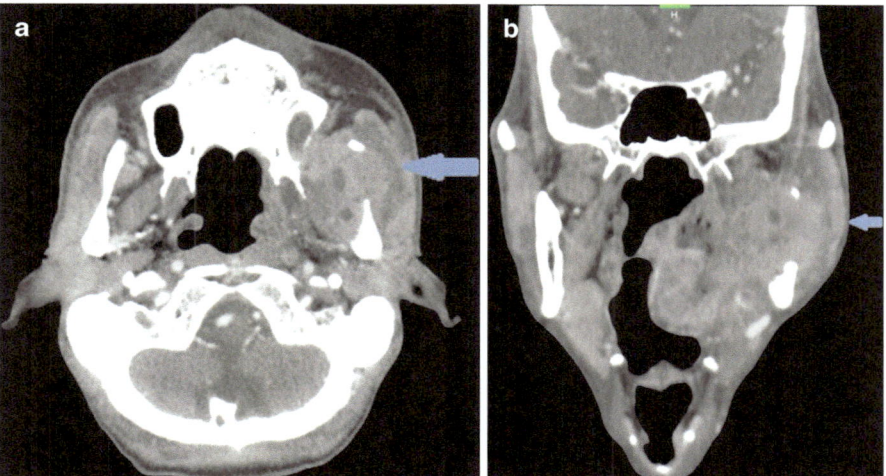

Fig. 2.10 T4 GB complex cancer (**a**) Showing invasion of infratemporal fossa. Note the loss of planes between pterygoid muscles and destruction of ascending ramus of mandible and upper alveolus (**b**) Coronal view of same patient

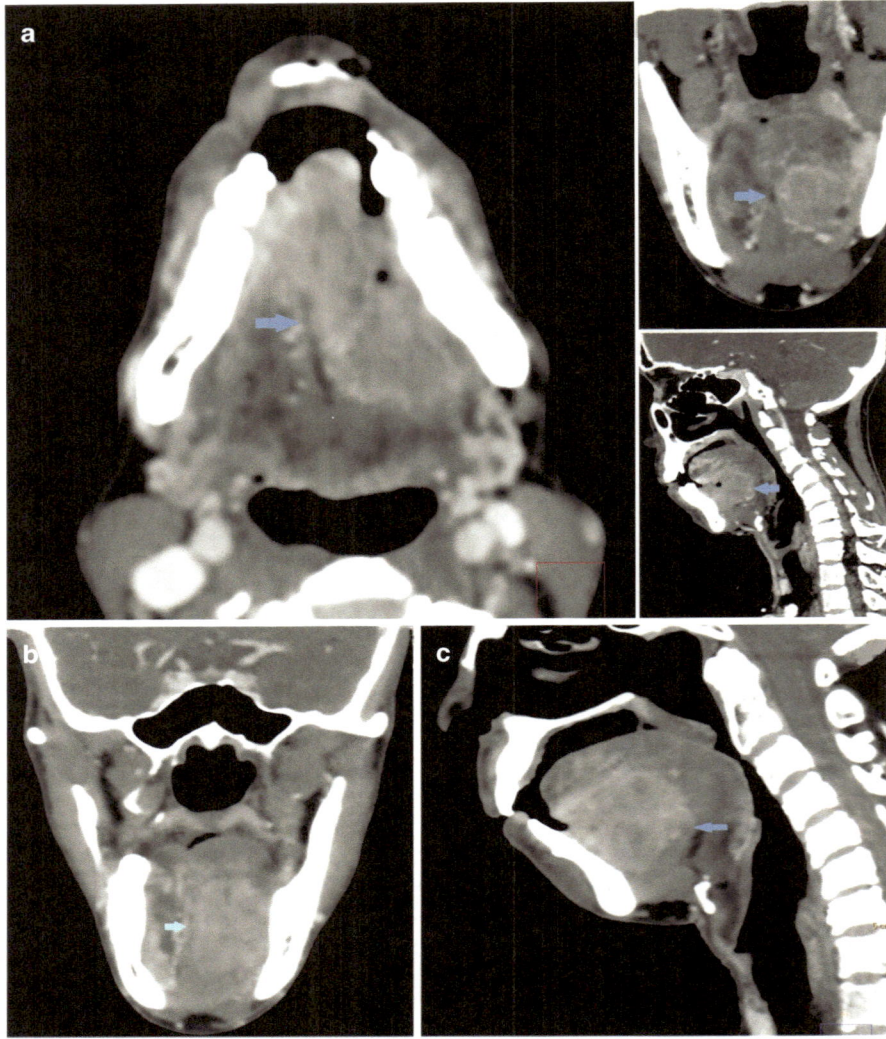

Fig. 2.11 (**a**) Advanced Ca tongue axial CT. (**b**) Advanced Ca tongue coronal CT of same patient. (**c**) Advanced Ca tongue sagittal CT of same patient

Fig. 2.12 Advanced Ca tongue MR axial (T1 non-contrast) showing mass involving right side tongue and large level II node

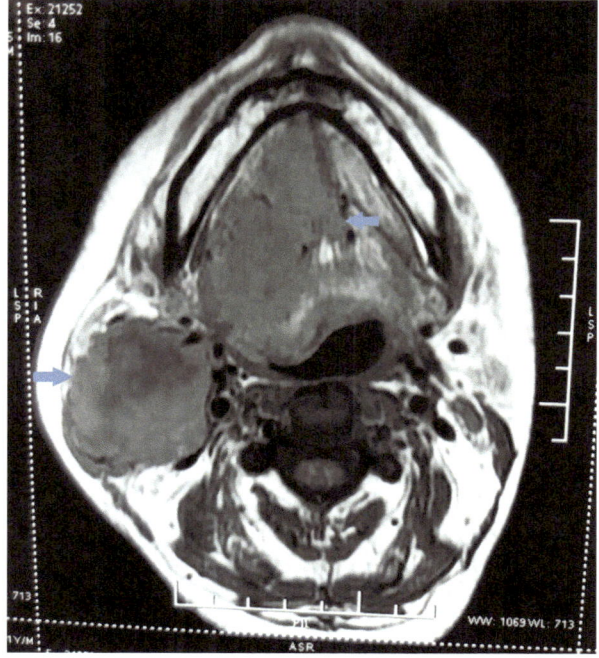

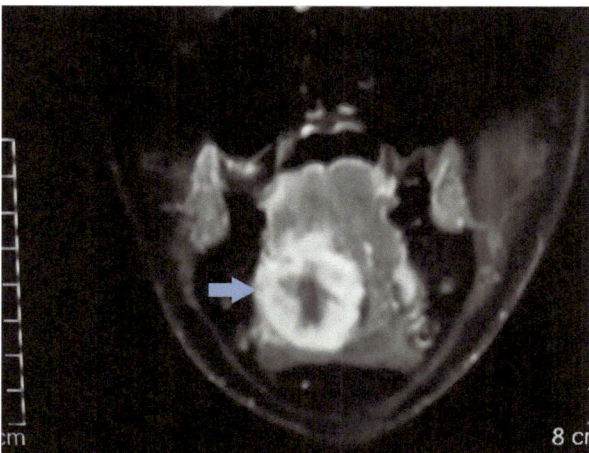

Fig. 2.13 Advanced Ca tongue Coronal MR with contrast showing T4 tumor extending into base tongue with involvement of extrinsic muscles of tongue

Fig. 2.14 Advanced Ca
tongue Sagittal T2 MR
clearly demonstrating
deeper extent of tumor
involvement

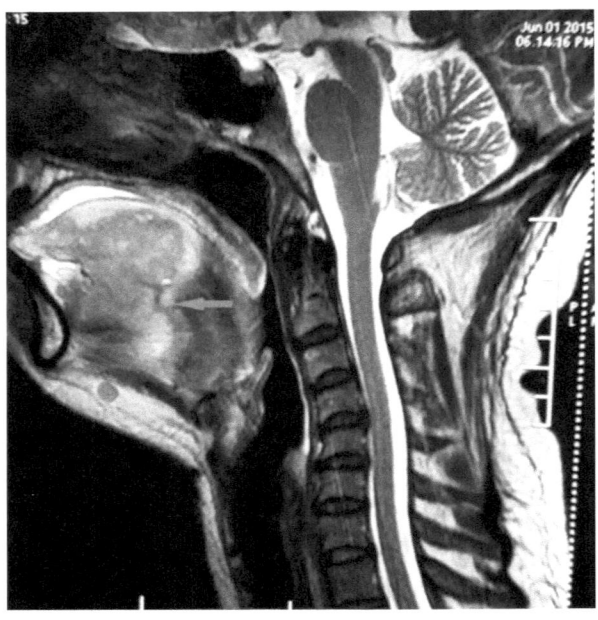

Oropharynx

3

Choice of Imaging

1. CT and MR both have equal merit for lesions involving tonsil/lateral pharyngeal wall.
2. In the case of posterior pharyngeal wall lesions, CT assesses bone invasion of vertebral body better though subtle involvement of prevertebral fascia may be better seen on MR.
3. Lesions of the base tongue are best assessed by MR to determine the depth of invasion.
4. Post-RT relapses are better assessed using PET-CT.

Pathology

1. While squamous cell Ca is the common pathology, it is important to consider minor salivary gland tumors (benign, malignant) in cases of submucosal lesions of the soft palate and base tongue.
2. For tonsillar lesions, the possibility of a lymphoma needs to be borne in mind.
3. Since the incidence of neck secondaries is high in oropharyngeal cancers, it is important to look for them during imaging.

© The Author(s) 2018

U. Nayak et al., *Clinical Radiology of Head and Neck Tumors*,
https://doi.org/10.1007/978-981-10-5036-7_3

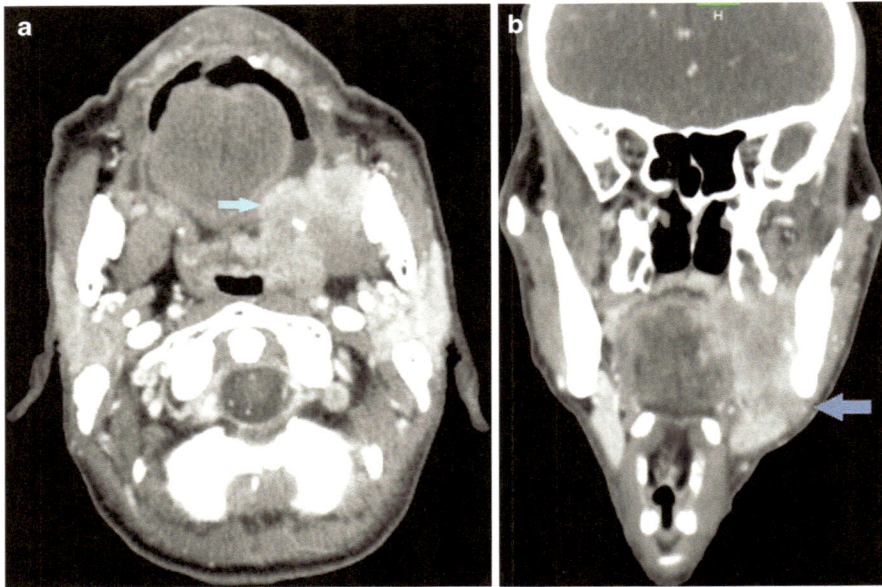

Fig. 3.1 (**a**) Ca Tonsil involving lateral pharyngeal wall and soft palate. (**b**) Ca tonsil extending to base tongue coronal CT reconstruction of same patient

Fig. 3.2 Ca oropharynx advanced disease with bilateral neck secondaries

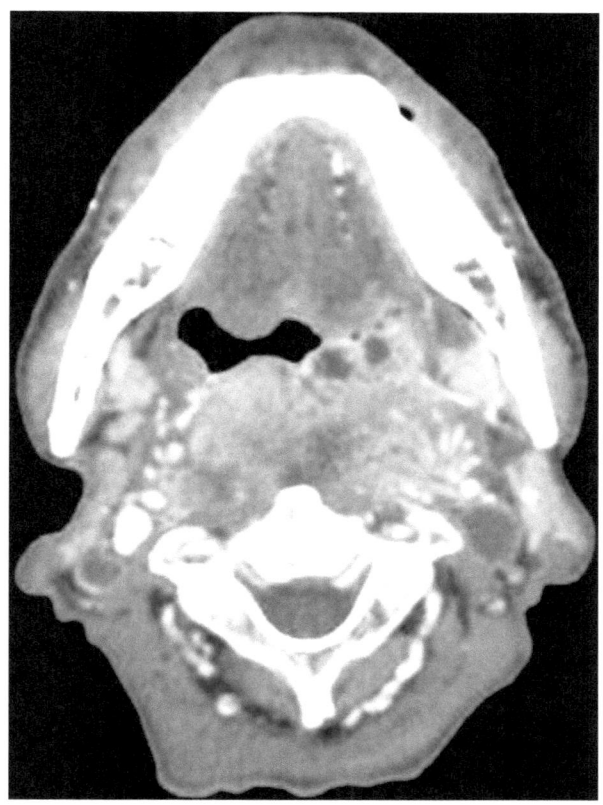

Fig. 3.3 Ca oropharynx advanced disease involving lateral and posterior pharyngeal wall and metastatic level 2 nodes

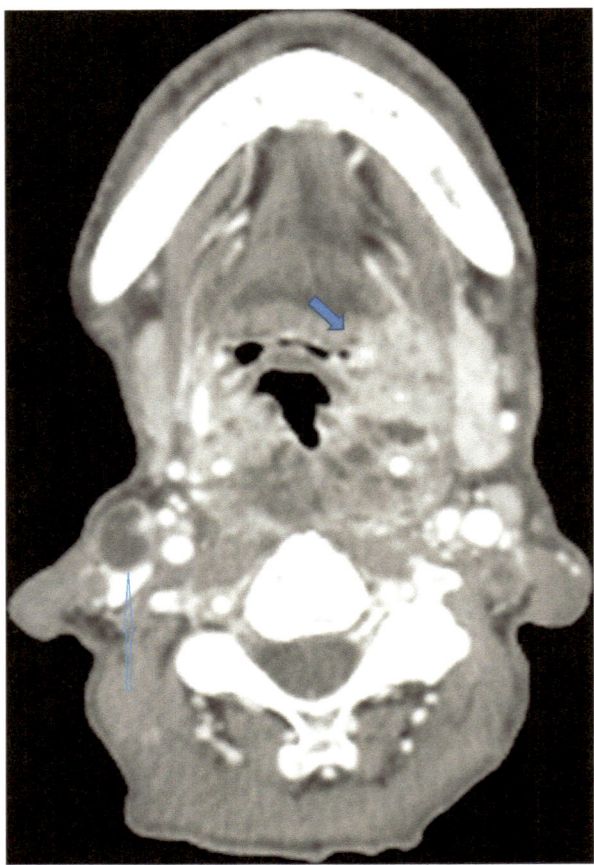

Fig. 3.4 Ca Oropharynx with vertebral body involvement. Axial CT suspicious for vertebral body involvement - to confirm with bone window

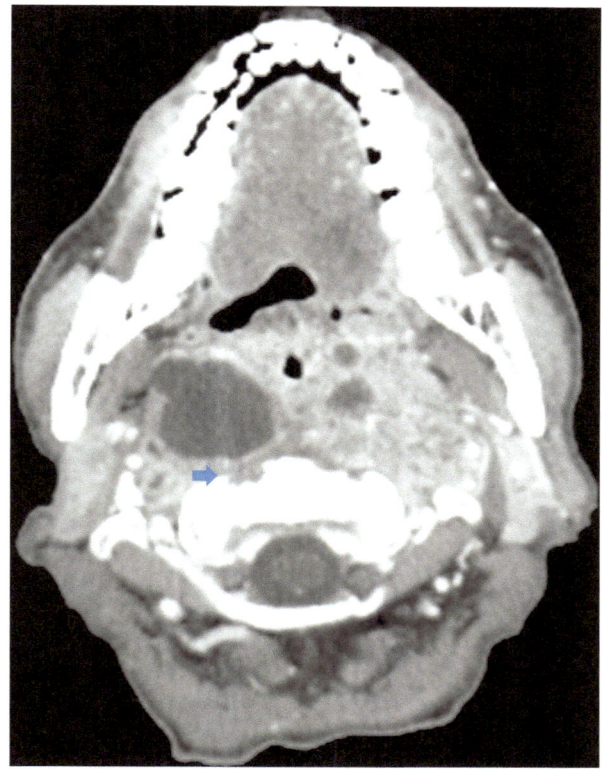

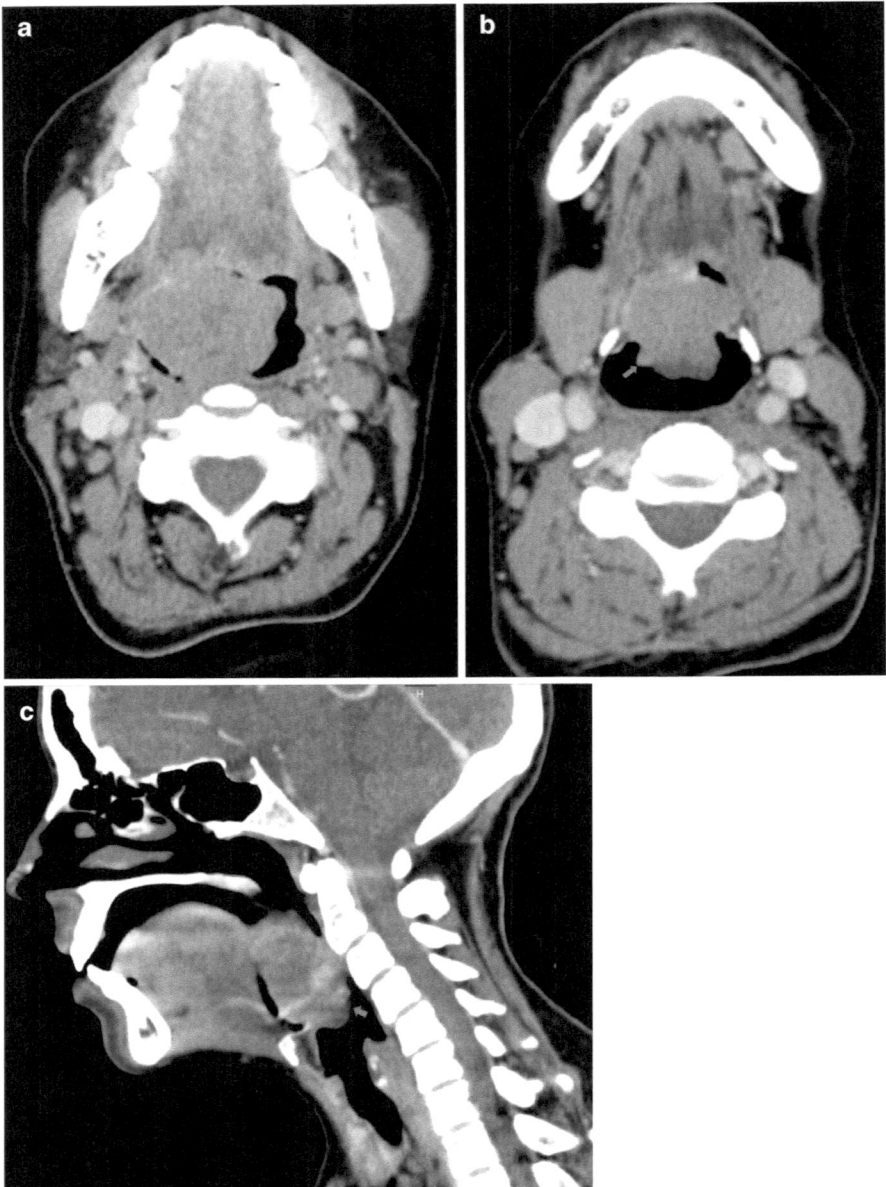

Fig. 3.5 (**a**) Minor salivary gland tumor arising from base tongue. (**b**) Minor salivary gland tumor showing extension into supraglottis. (**c**) Minor salivary gland tumor sagittal CT of same patient

Fig. 3.6 Minor salivary gland tumor sagittal CT

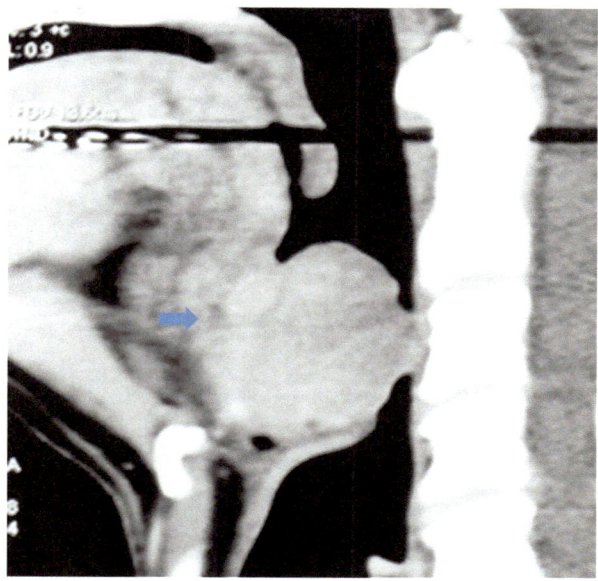

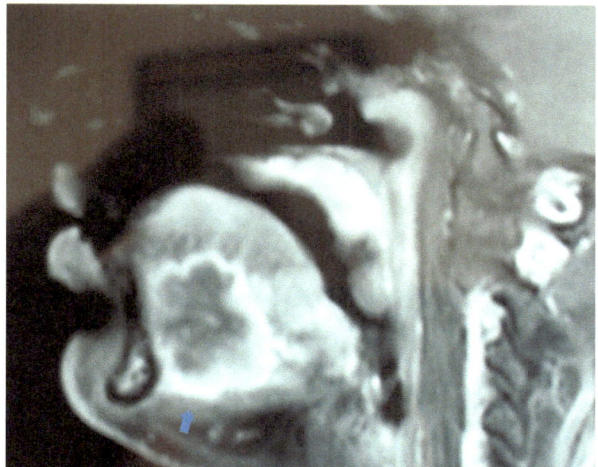

Fig. 3.7 Ca base tongue sagittal MR (T1 contrast) demonstrating clearly depth of infiltration of the base of tongue

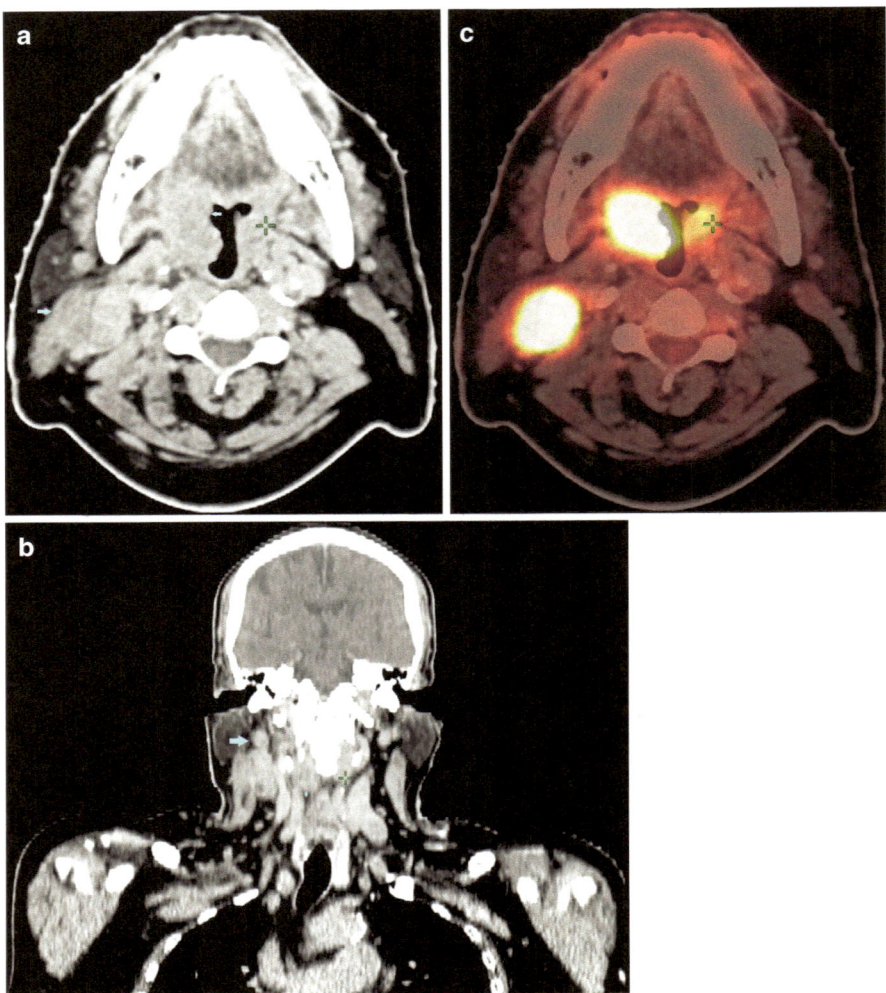

Fig. 3.8 (**a**) MUO right level II. CT revealed primary in right tonsil (artifact over left tonsil). (**b**) MUO right level II with primary in tonsil. CT coronal reconstruction. (**c**) MUO right level II with primary in tonsil PET-CT (left tonsil showing physiological uptake)

Choice of Imaging

1. **HRCT** (High resolution CT) with thin (2 mm) cuts has been the imaging modality of choice for early laryngeal cancer.
2. **MR** was traditionally used more for problem-solving in difficult situations; however in recent times, MR has established itself as a useful tool in the evaluation of early cancers, especially when deciding between trans-oral laser excision versus external radiation as treatment modality.
3. In advanced cancers, CT is generally preferred to assess cartilage involvement and extra-laryngeal spread.
4. MR scores over CT in assessing both subclinical nodal disease and to visualize the character of larger nodes to help differentiate metastatic involvement from reactive changes.

In Early Cancers

1. Laryngoscopy provides the initial assessment of the disease status, the extent of mucosal involvement, and vocal cord mobility while imaging helps upstage the disease by providing information regarding pre-epiglottic/paraglottic/subglottic extensions and status of thyroid cartilage as well as the presence of subclinical neck secondaries.
2. In cancer involving anterior commissure, imaging can upstage disease status from T1 to T4 (thyroid cartilage involvement) a finding which may be missed on clinical examination.

© The Author(s) 2018   31
U. Nayak et al., *Clinical Radiology of Head and Neck Tumors*,
https://doi.org/10.1007/978-981-10-5036-7_4

In Advanced Cancer

1. Paraglottic spread of disease (indicating a T3 transglottic cancer) which may be missed on laryngoscopy can be clearly demonstrated by contrast CT/MR.
2. Imaging can aid in the accurate assessment of the extent of disease by demonstrating cartilage destruction, soft tissue spread (thyroid gland/strap muscles), and carotid encasement—indicating inoperability (T4b).
3. In post-RT status, CT has a limited role in differentiating edema/fibrosis from disease relapse. MR by DWI (diffusion weighted imaging) scores over CT, but PET-CT is the generally preferred imaging modality in this situation.

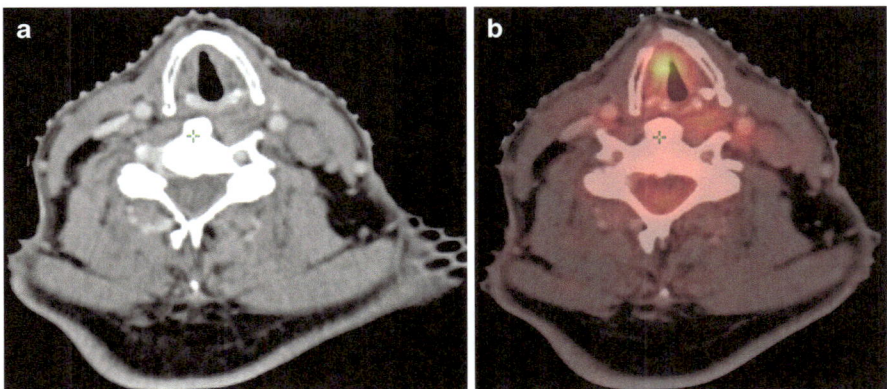

Fig. 4.1 (**a**) Glottic Ca T1 stage (*right vocal cord*) axial CT showing no obvious abnormality. (Artifact on vertebral body). (**b**) Glottic Ca T1 stage PET-CT of same patient demonstrating right vocal cord lesion

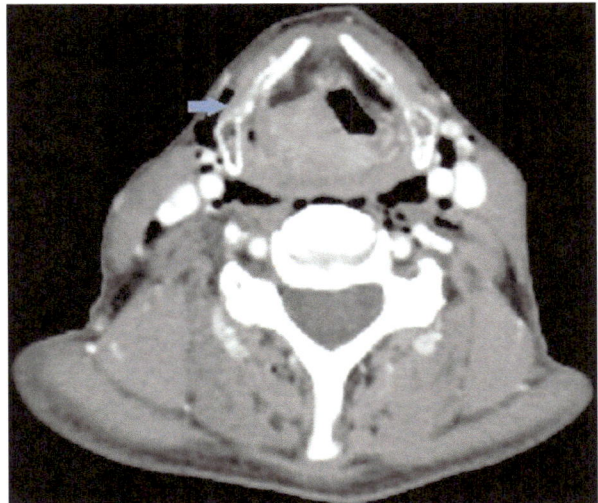

Fig. 4.2 Glottic cancer T3 stage axial CT at false cord level showing tumor involving paraglottic space and inter-arytenoid area

Fig. 4.3 Glottic cancer T3
stage axial CT at level of
glottis showing paraglottic
spread of cancer

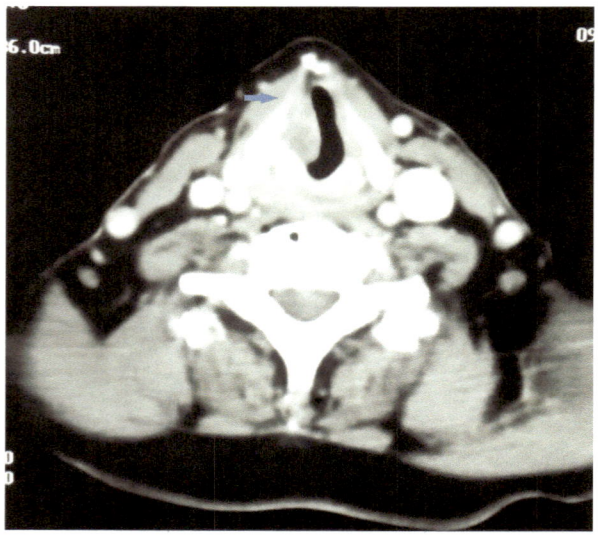

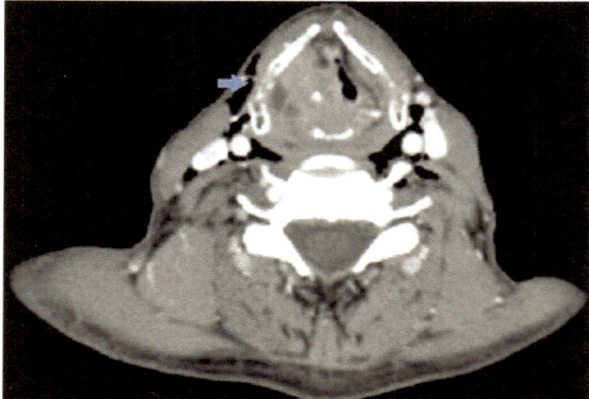

Fig. 4.4 Glottic cancer T3
axial CT at the level of
glottis with cartilage
invovement, not penetrated
through and through
cartilage

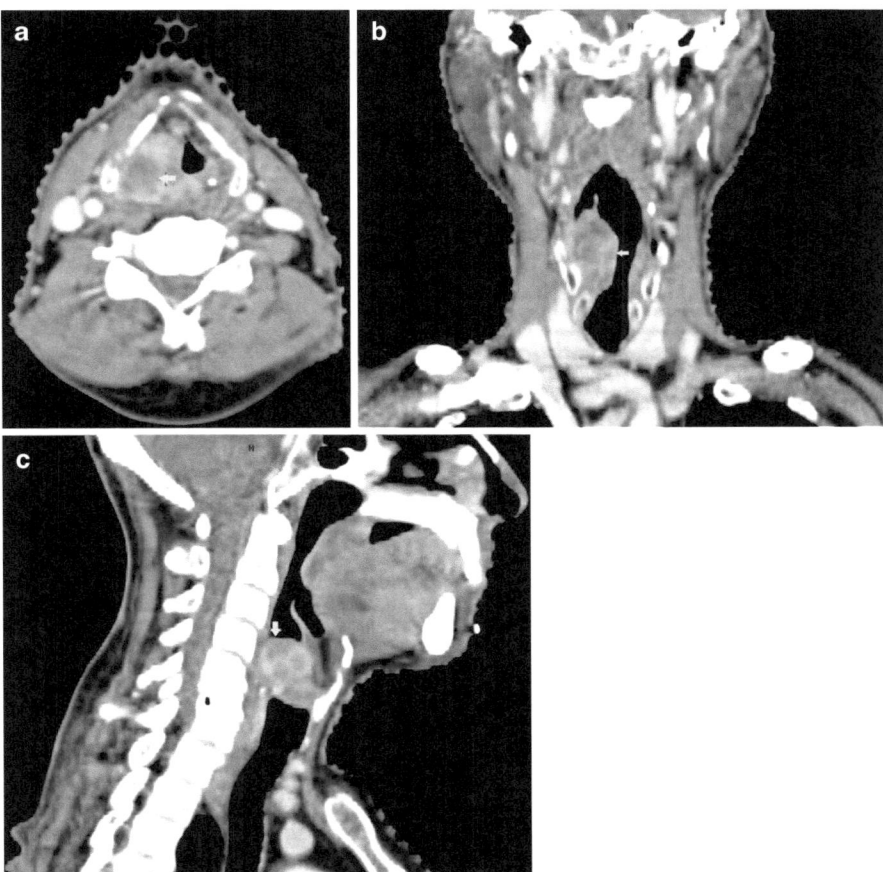

Fig. 4.5 (a) Ca larynx T4 axial CT demonstrating cartilage destruction penetrating through and through. (b) Ca larynx T4 coronal reconstruction to demonstrate subglottic extension and transglottic spread. (c) Transglottic Ca T4 sagittal images

Fig. 4.6 Glottic cancer T4
axial CT showing gross
cartilage destruction and
soft tissue extension

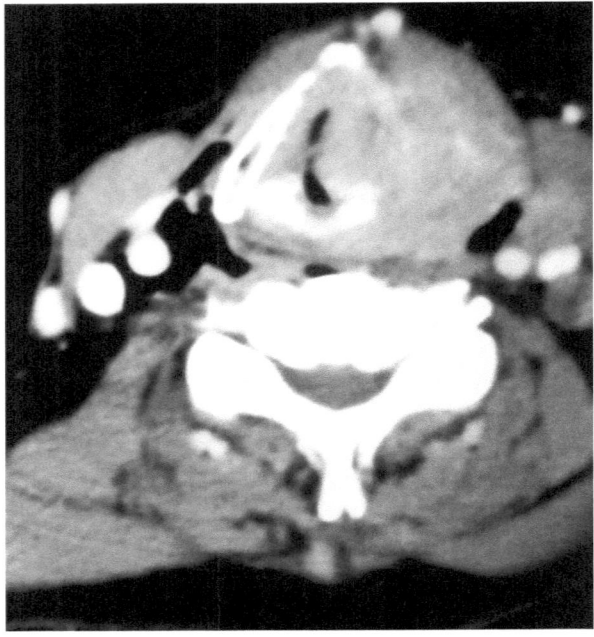

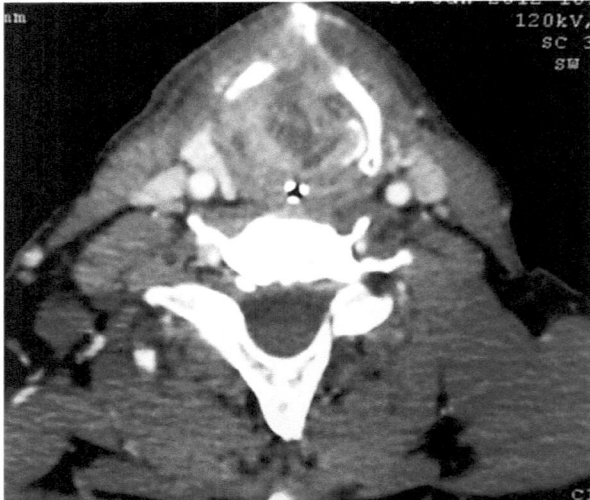

Fig. 4.7 Advanced
laryngeal cancer axial CT
showing cartilage
destruction and total
obliteration of laryngeal
lumen. Note Ryle's tube
in situ

Fig. 4.8 Recurrent glottic cancer post CTRT PET-CT scan

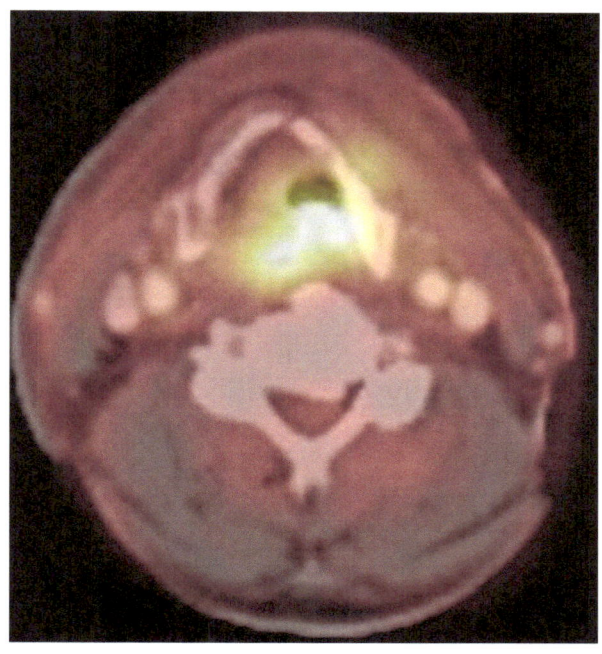

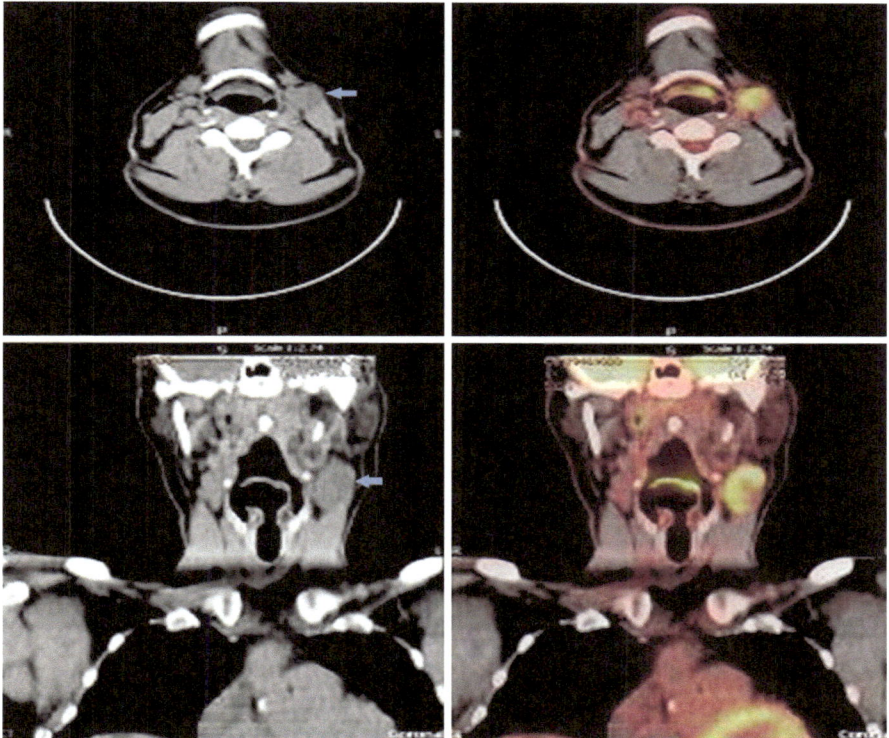

Fig. 4.9 MUO neck CT showed only neck node, PET-CT was able to identify early T1 primary over epiglottis not recognized on laryngoscopy

Fig. 4.10 (**a**) Paraganglioma larynx right side—
CT axial notice the intense
enhancement. (**b**)
Paraganglioma larynx
coronal reconstruction of
same patient

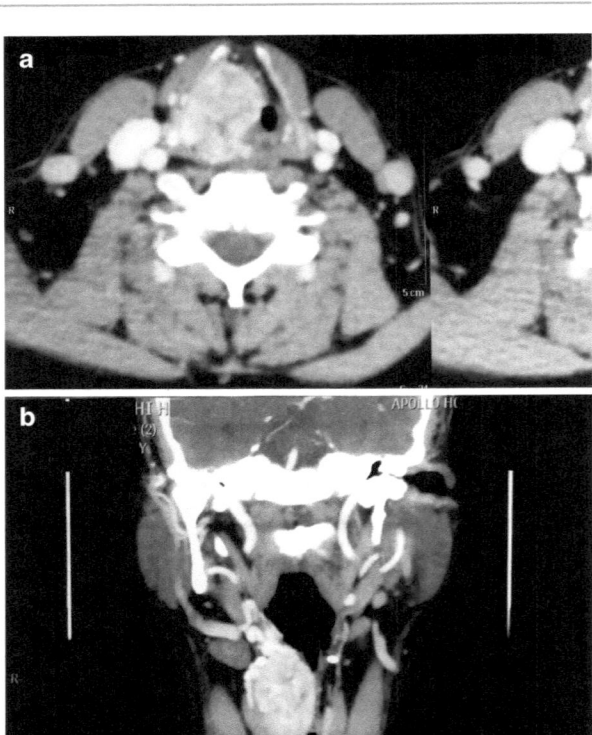

Hypopharynx

5

Choice of Imaging

1. **MR** is generally preferred in early and moderately advanced hypopharyngeal cancer.
2. **CT** delineates cartilage and vertebral body invasion better in advanced cases.
3. **PET-CT** is the best modality for assessing disease status following chemoradiation though it may also be utilized to rule out distant metastasis in advanced cases especially in those presenting with bulky nodal disease.

In Early Cancer

1. Imaging by itself has limited role in the assessment of primary disease and needs to be correlated with endoscopy findings, but MR is of value in assessing subclinical neck disease and in disease staging.
2. Often PET-CT may identify small volume disease better rather than CT or MR.

In Advanced Cancer

1. Vocal cord fixity is a clinical finding and may not be appreciated generally on imaging though paramedian position of the cord may give some clue.
2. Imaging (CT or MR) is mandatory for accurate staging of the disease as well as for determination of operability. Retropharyngeal node involvement, prevertebral invasion, carotid encasement, and mediastinal extension may preclude surgery.
3. Though imaging will help determine surgical operability, exact extent of surgery and choice of reconstructive options may only be decided during endoscopy/surgery.

© The Author(s) 2018   39
U. Nayak et al., *Clinical Radiology of Head and Neck Tumors*,
https://doi.org/10.1007/978-981-10-5036-7_5

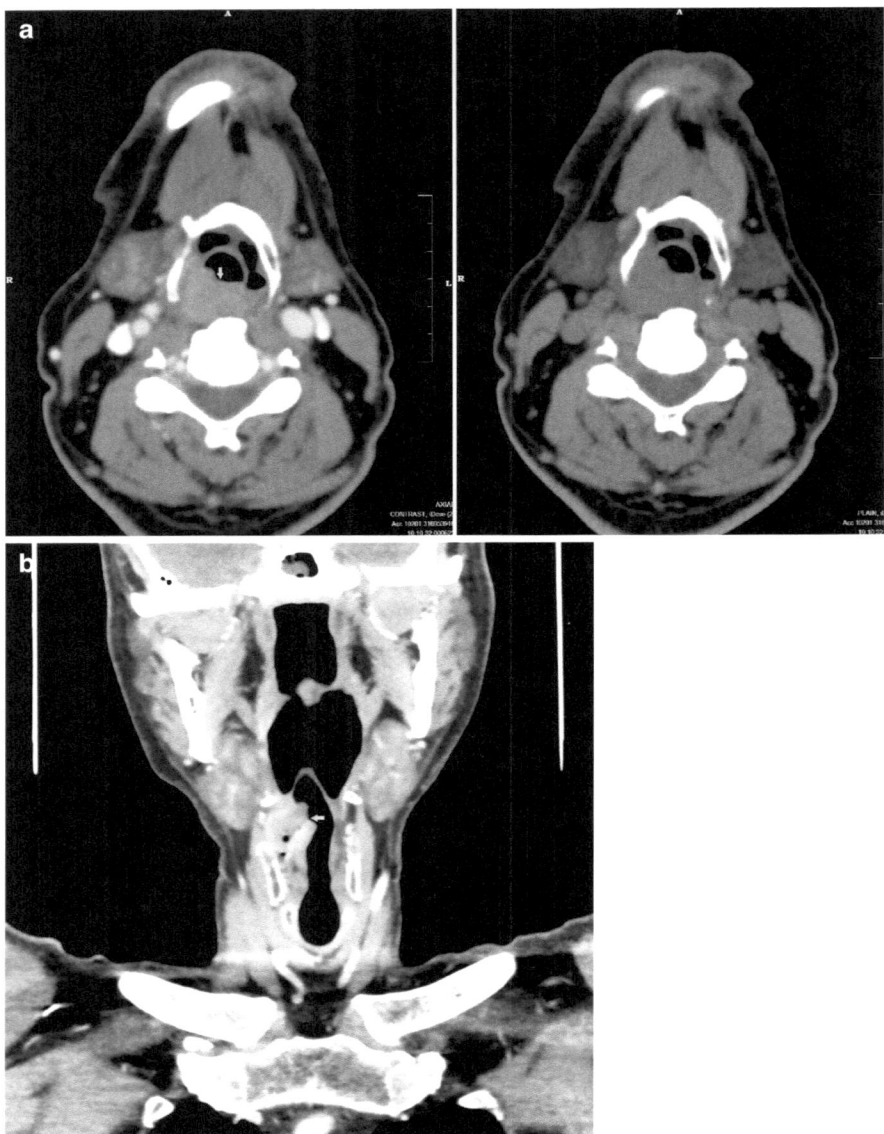

Fig. 5.1 (**a**) Ca pyriform sinus T2 involving AE fold—axial CT contrast enhanced (*left*) and plain (*right*). (**b**) Ca pyriform sinus T2 involving AE fold—coronal reconstruction of same patient

Fig. 5.2 (**a**) Ca pyriform sinus T2 stage involving AE fold MR axial T1 sequence. (**b**) Ca pyriform sinus MR axial T2 sequence of same patient. (**c**) Ca pyriform sinus T2 stage axial MR STIR (same patient)

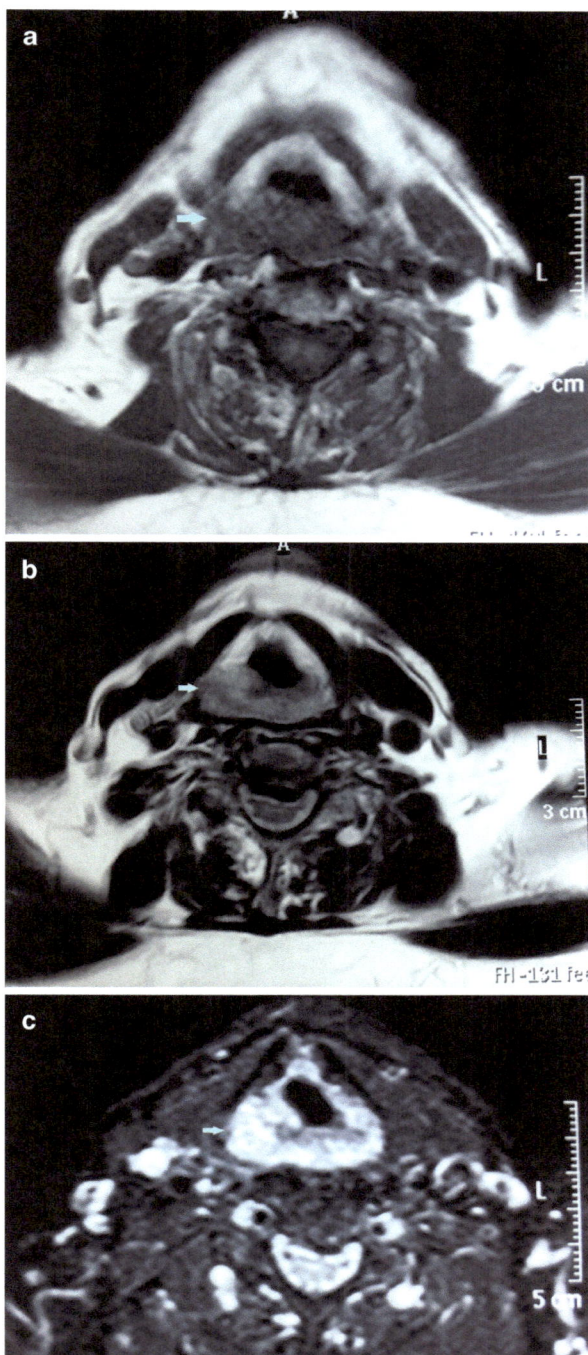

Fig. 5.3 (**a**) Ca pyriform
sinus T2 stage PET-CT.
(**b**) Ca pyriform sinus
PET-CT coronal
reconstruction of same
patient

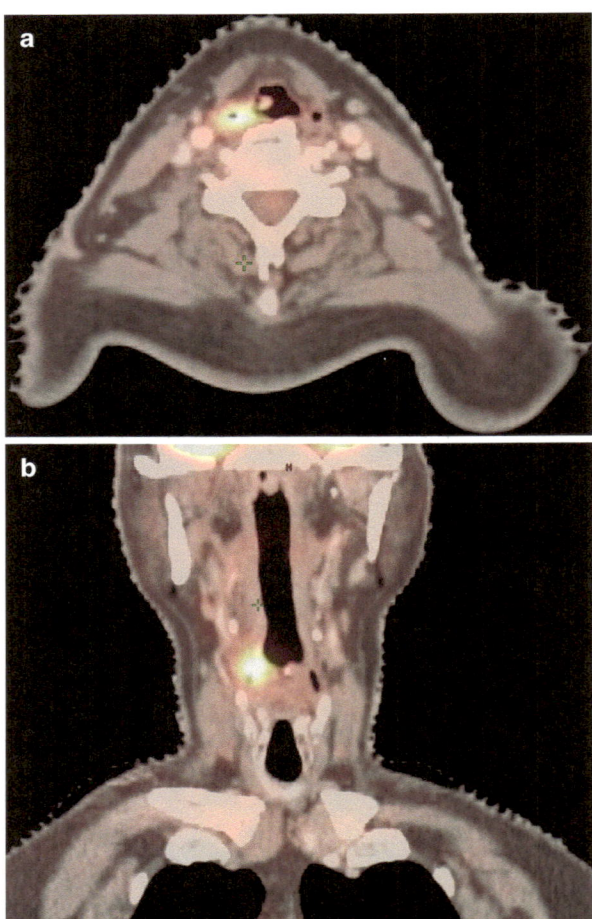

Fig. 5.4 Ca hypopharynx
T3 stage axial CT
showing extension
into supraglottis—pre-
epiglottic space is not
involved

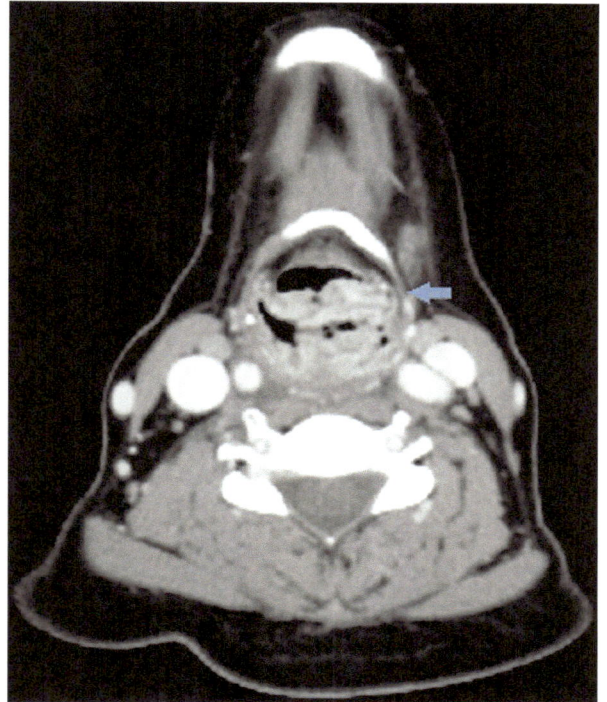

Fig. 5.5 (**a**) Ca pyriform sinus T3 stage axial CT with involvement of lateral and posterior pharyngeal wall. (**b**) Pyriform sinus T3 same patient showing that apex of PFS is uninvolved

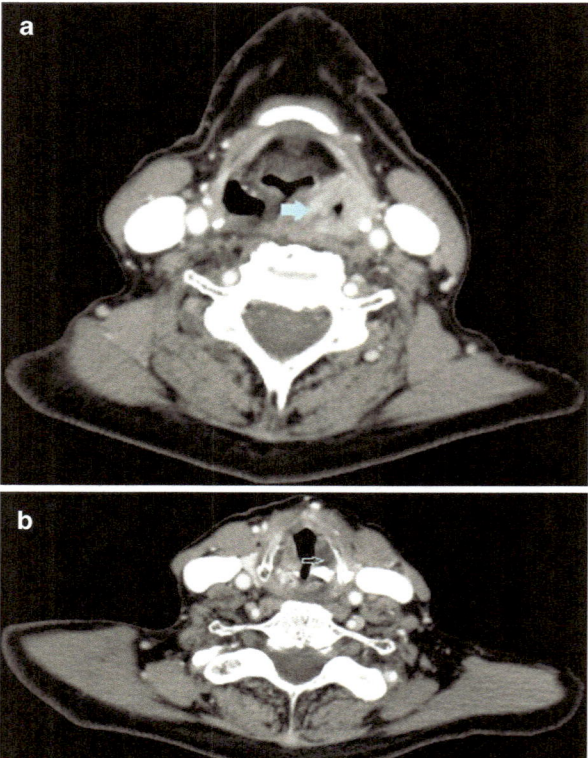

Fig. 5.6 Post CTRT Ca
hypopharynx with gross
laryngeal oedema

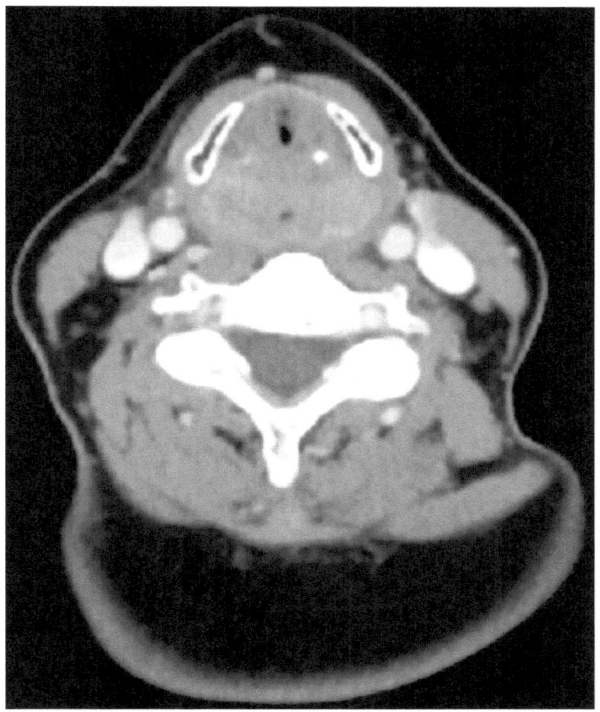

Fig. 5.7 (**a**) Ca post
cricoid with near-total
luminal obstruction—axial
CT. (**b**) Ca Post cricoid
axial CT chest of same
patient showing tumor
extending into cervical
oesophagus – will require
total oesophagectomy
along with
laryngo-pharyngectomy

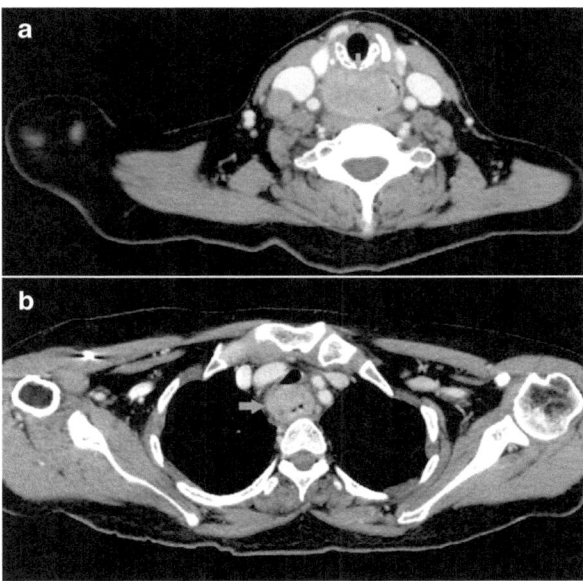

Fig. 5.8 Ca hypopharynx
with retropharyngeal node

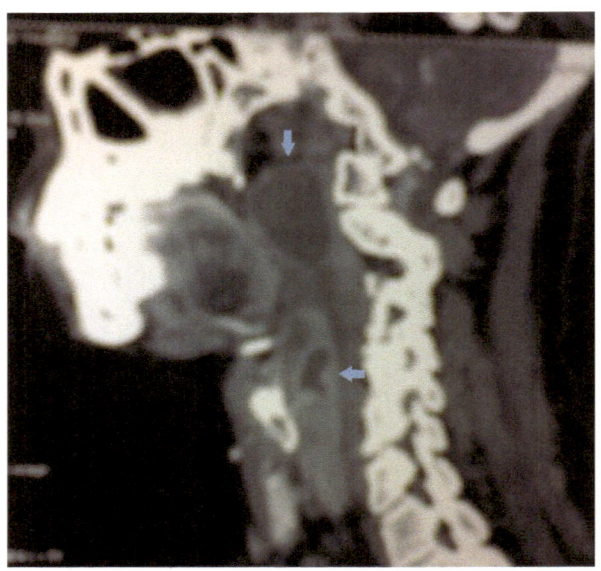

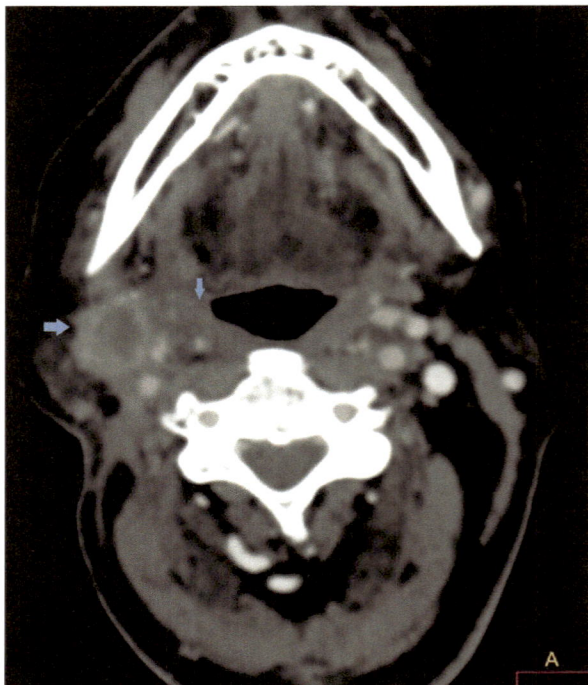

Fig. 5.9 Ca pyriform
sinus post RT Axial CT
showing residual primary
and node

Fig. 5.10 Ca posterior
pharyngeal wall axial CT

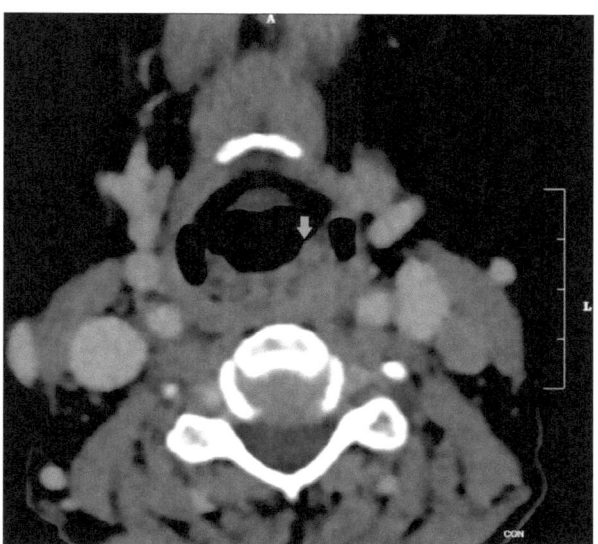

Neck

6

Choice of Imaging

Cervical Lymphadenopathy

1. **USG** plays an important role in the detection of subclinical neck nodes (inflammatory or neoplastic). The ease and wide availability of this modality makes it the natural choice for initial evaluation.
2. **CT and MR** are generally preferred for the assessment of advanced neck disease (both inflammatory and neoplastic).
3. Additional advantage of CT and MR in a suspected case of metastatic cervical lymphadenopathy is to aid in the detection of a possible primary.
4. **PET-CT** is more sensitive and preferred in the evaluation of metastasis from unknown primary (MUO). It is also the preferred modality in post-CTRT and postsurgical nodal relapse to differentiate recurrence from fibrosis and in the staging of lymphomas.

Soft Tissue Tumors

MR scores over CT for soft tissue delineation and to identify possible tissue of origin (nerve, muscle, fat, lymphatic, etc.).

Lymphovascular Malformations

MR is again the preferred choice of imaging in lymphovascular malformation to differentiate between lymphangioma, hemangioma, and A-V malformation. MR (T1 contrast) demonstrates cystic spaces with wall enhancement in lymphangioma, a hyperintense signal in A-V malformation with flow voids in T2 and cystic spaces with phleboliths in case of cavernous haemangioma.

© The Author(s) 2018
U. Nayak et al., *Clinical Radiology of Head and Neck Tumors*,
https://doi.org/10.1007/978-981-10-5036-7_6

Points to Note

1. In metastatic cervical lymphadenopathy, the possible site of primary also needs to be looked at during imaging (CT/MR); the level and location of the nodal disease can give an indication as to where the primary disease could be arising from:
   (a) Level I—oral cavity
   (b) Level II—any site in the upper aerodigestive tract, PNS, or salivary gland
   (c) Level III–IV—larynx, hypopharynx, cervical esophagus, thyroid
   (d) Level V—nasopharynx (upper level V nodes), thyroid, and infraclavicular primary (lower level V nodes)
2. CT/MR can sometimes aid in differentiating the possible pathology (TB, lymphoma, metastasis) based on certain characteristics—such as shape of the nodes (rounded in metastasis and oval in inflammatory), perinodal infiltration and the presence of central necrosis in metastasis, discrete and fleshy without necrosis in lymphomas and the presence of caseation and cold abscess in TB. FNAC/biopsy is generally required for confirmation.
3. Imaging is mandatory to determine operability of any neck mass. Involvement of vascular structures, fixity to underlying structures (prevertebral muscles, spine, base of skull, etc.) can be appreciated in CT/MR.

Fig. 6.1 TB cervical lymphadenopathy CT axial showing caseation necrosis

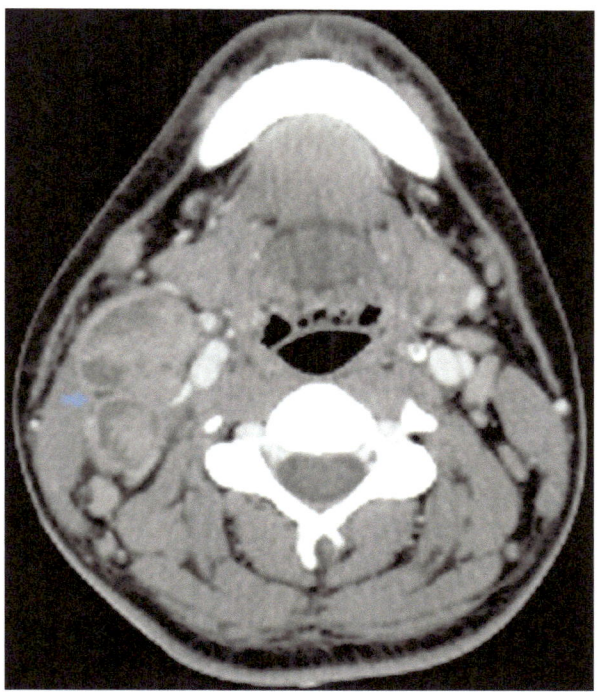

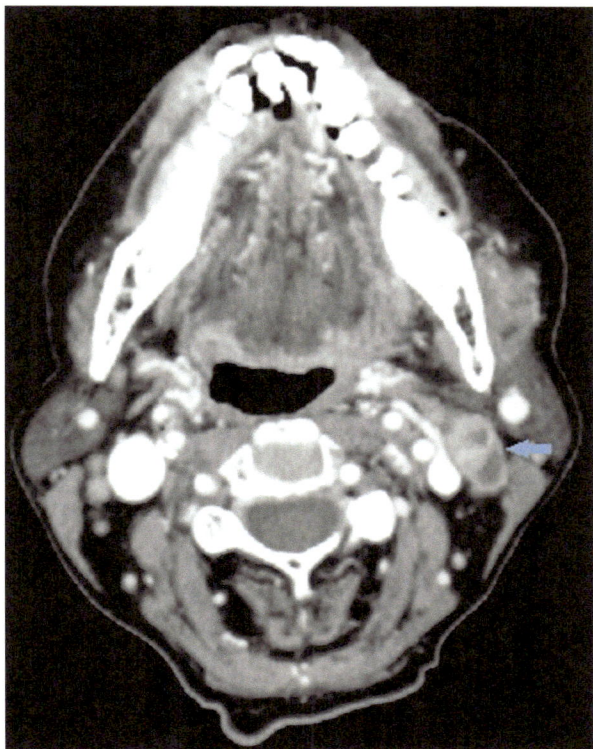

Fig. 6.2 Neck secondaries metastatic level II node showing central necrosis and rounded shape with perinodal thickening and compression of IJV

Fig. 6.3 (a) Neck secondaries CT axial showing large metastatic node in upper posterior triangle. (b) Upper cuts of same patient demonstrating nasopharyngeal mass suggestive of Ca nasopharynx

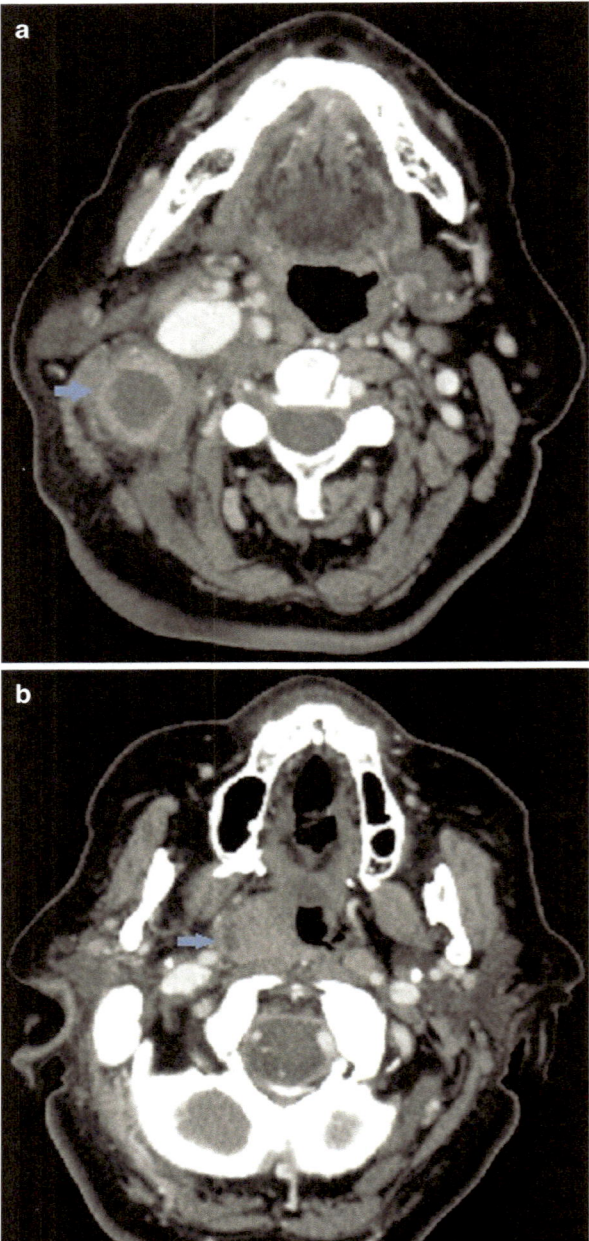

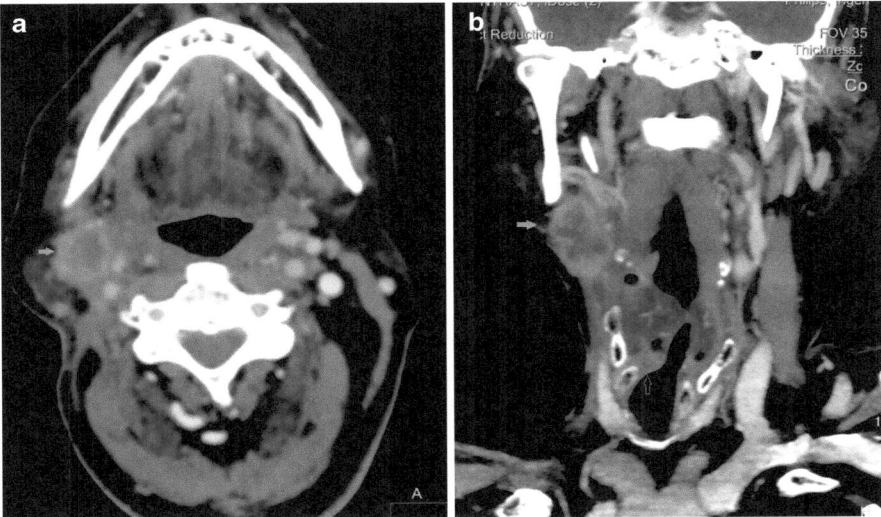

Fig. 6.4 (**a**) Neck secondaries post CTRT Ca hypopharynx with residual neck node disease. Central necrosis with indistinct borders. (**b**) Coronal reconstruction showing primary in hypopharynx (*hollow arrow*)

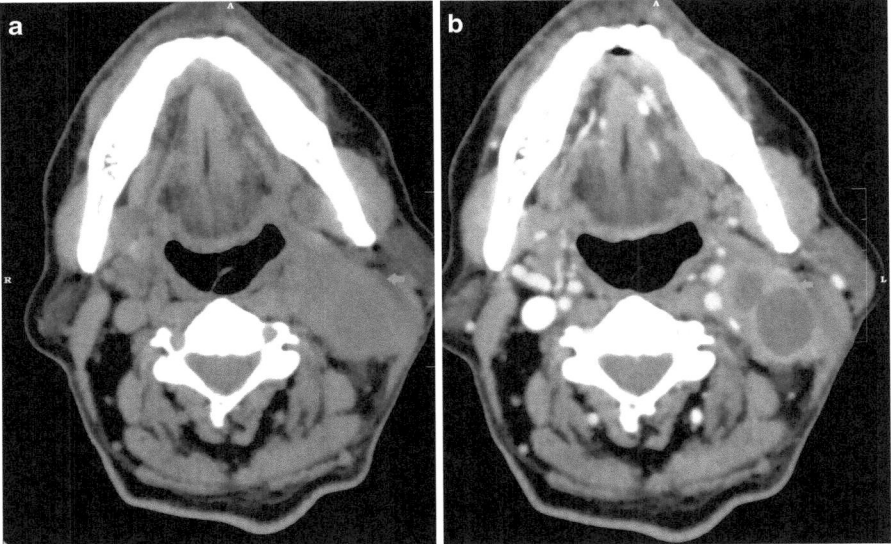

Fig. 6.5 Branchial cyst (**a**) pre-contrast and (**b**) post-contrast CT

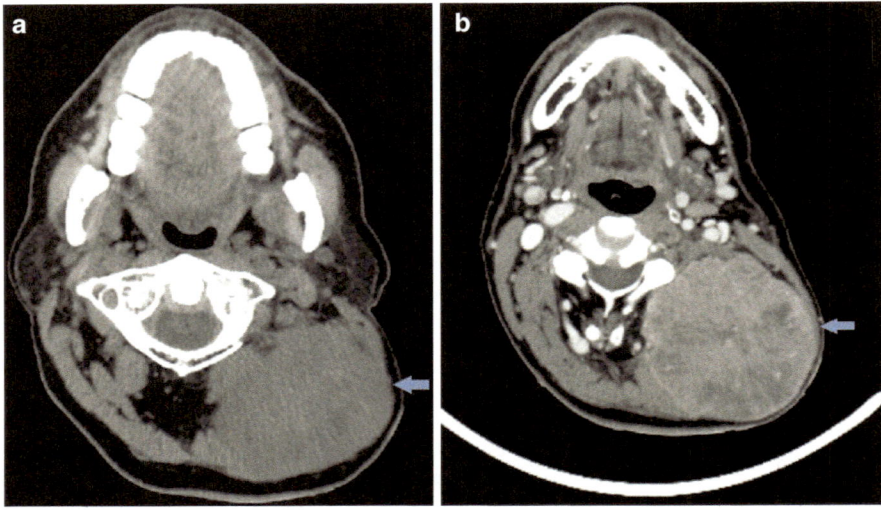

Fig. 6.6 (a) Soft tissue tumor axial CT posterior neck mass (plain CT). (b) Post contrast study of same patient

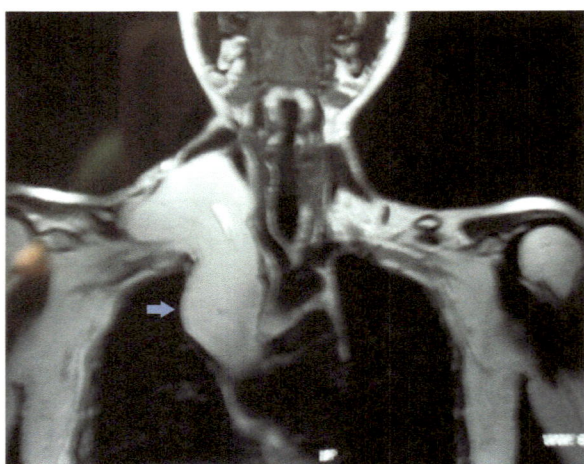

Fig. 6.7 Lipoma lower neck. Coronal MR showing extension into superior mediastinum

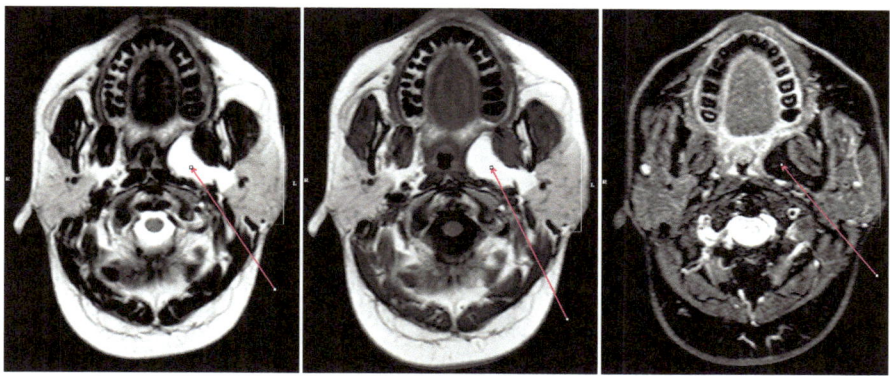

Fig. 6.8 Lipoma neck axial MR: T2, T1 and STIR

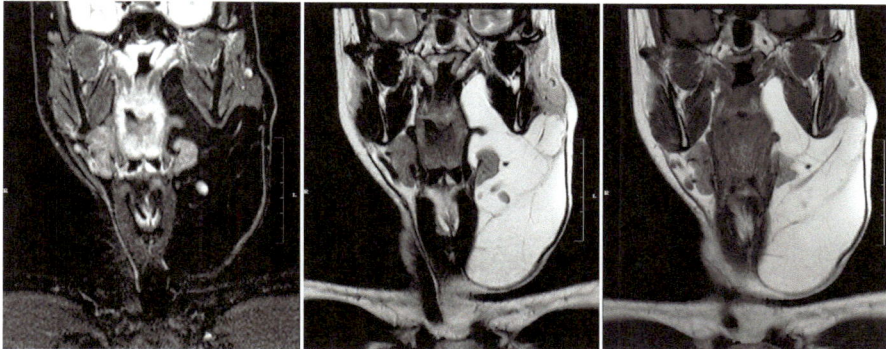

Fig. 6.9 Lipoma neck coronal MR: STIR, T2, T1

Fig. 6.10 Neurofibroma
MR neck showing tumor
arising from cervical
plexus

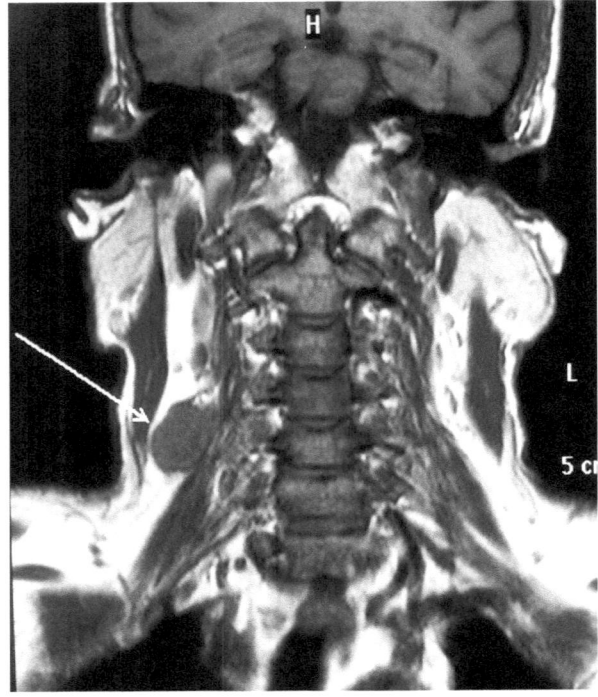

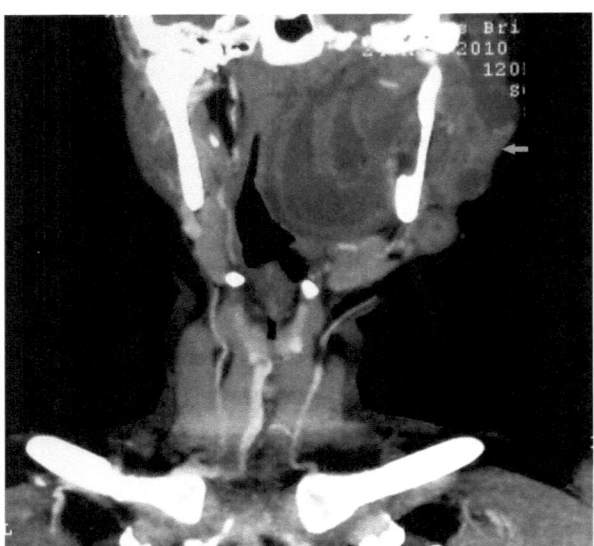

Fig. 6.11 Multiple
neurofibromas coronal CT

Choice of Imaging

Thyroid

1. **Ultrasound** is the preferred imaging modality in the initial evaluation of all thyroid nodules and helps evaluate:
   (a) Size, location, and number of nodules and their characteristics (cystic, solid, mixed)
   (b) Status of opposite lobe to differentiate solitary nodule from multinodular goiter. This will aid in risk stratification for malignancy
   (c) For guided FNAC in non-palpable nodules as well as to direct the needle to representative area (solid component) in palpable nodules
   (d) Presence of metastatic cervical nodes in malignancies
   (e) Monitor progression of benign nodules in patients kept on observation
   (f) Follow up post-thyroidectomy in Ca thyroid
   (g) During evaluation of metastatic papillary carcinoma in patients presenting with cervical lymphadenopathy with no detectable primary to identify the presence of any thyroid nodule and possible primary.
2. **Technetium thyroid scan** is indicated in the evaluation of patients with hyperthyroidism. Grave's disease shows diffuse high uptake throughout the gland, toxic nodule shows increased uptake in the nodule (hot nodule) and reduced uptake in rest of the gland and toxic MNG shows increased uptake in internodular areas with reduced uptake in the nodules (cold nodules).
3. **CT/MR** is not indicated in routine evaluation of thyroid swelling but is mandatory to confirm substernal extension, tracheal/vascular compression in locally invasive thyroid malignancies and in the evaluation of the superior medistinum in medullary carcinomas. In the evaluation of very large benign nodules where trachea is not palpable, CT may help identify involved lobe and guide surgery. It is important to remember that CT may miss subclinical thyroid nodules which may often be picked up on USG. CT is also useful in the evaluation of recurrent thyroid cancer.

© The Author(s) 2018
U. Nayak et al., *Clinical Radiology of Head and Neck Tumors*,
https://doi.org/10.1007/978-981-10-5036-7_7

4. **Radioactive iodine scan** is used in the postsurgery follow-up of Ca thyroid while CT/PET-CT is reserved for patients with rising thyroglobulin levels and normal USG and RAI scan.
5. **PET-CT scan** may be indicated in evaluation of dedifferentiated, non-radioiodine avid recurrent thyroid cancers.

Parathyroid

1. **USG** is the preferred modality for identification and localization of enlarged parathyroid.
2. **Sestamibi scan** may also be used for localization. In the initial phase both thyroid and parathyroid take up the isotope, in delayed images there is a washout from the thyroid but the abnormal parathyroid gland retains the dye.
3. **SPECT** may help localize parathyroid enlargement in cases where USG findings may be equivocal.
4. **CT** is reserved for parathyroid Ca to look for infiltration to surrounding structures. 4-D CT is one of the recent advances in parathyroid imaging which can give information about the approx weight of the enlarged parathyroid in addition to improved localization to facilitate focused minimally invasive parathyroidectomy.

Fig. 7.1 Colloid cyst—larger one *right lobe* and small one *left lobe*

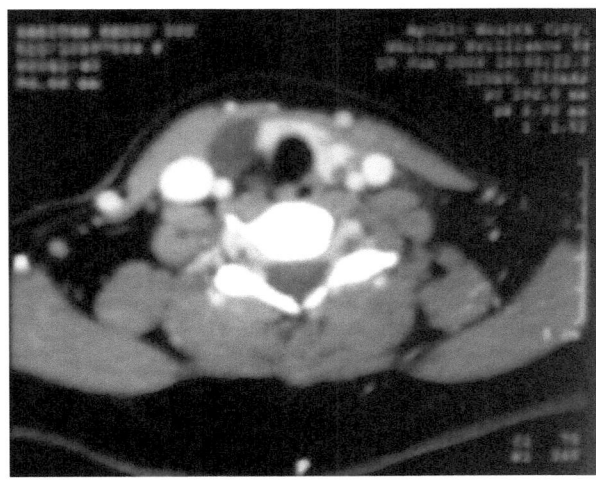

Fig. 7.2 Multinodular goitre involving both thyroid lobes

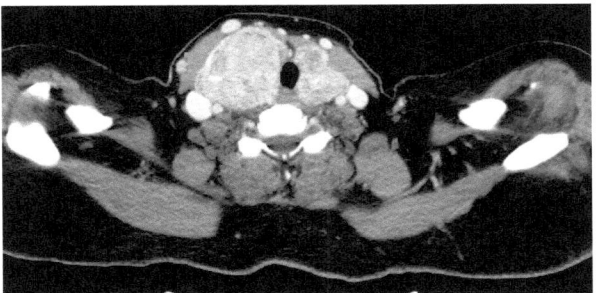

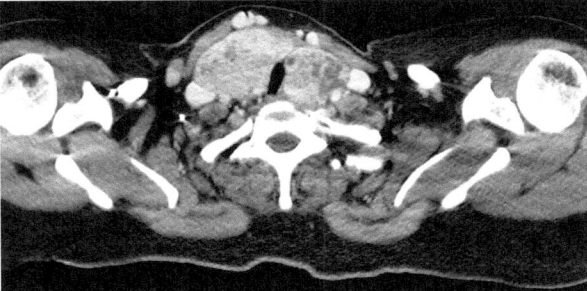

Fig. 7.3 Multinodular goitre causing tracheal compression (scabbard trachea)

Fig. 7.4 (**a**) Substernal
goitre causing tracheal
compression. (**b**)
Substernal goitre—coronal
reconstruction of same
patient

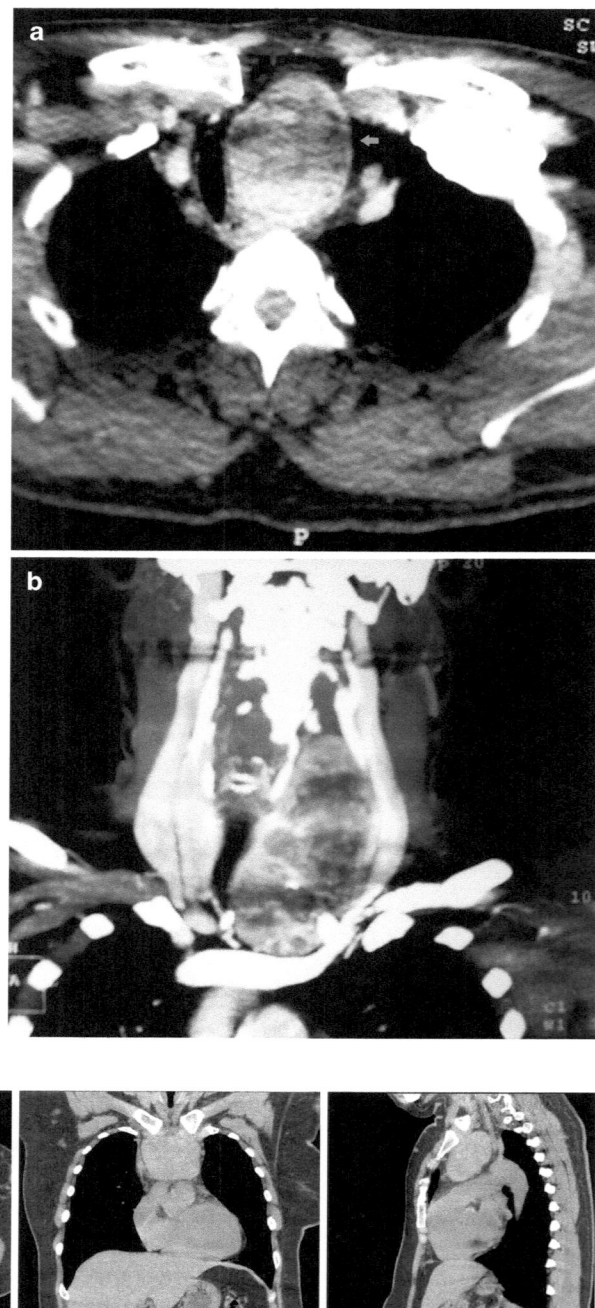

Fig. 7.5 Substernal goitre—CT axial, coronal, sagittal

Fig. 7.6 Substernal goitre both thyroid lobes showing substernal extension

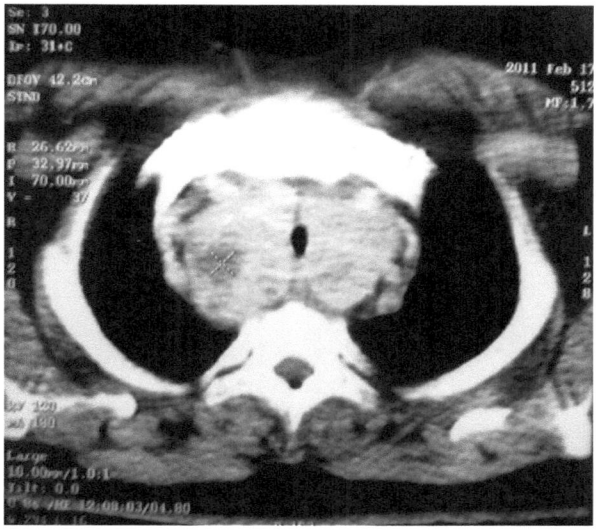

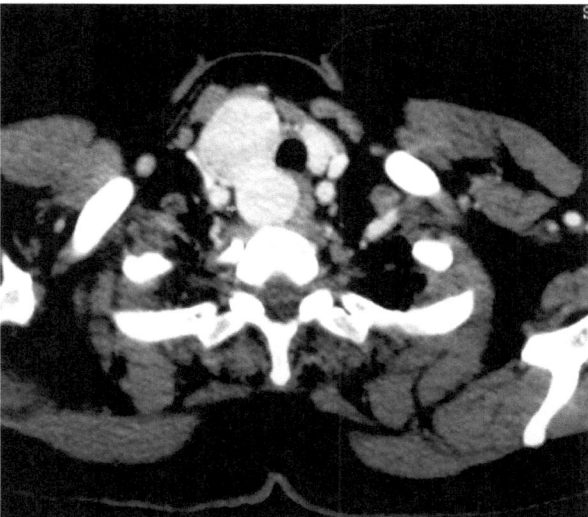

Fig. 7.7 Retro-tracheal goitre - higher risk of injury to RLN

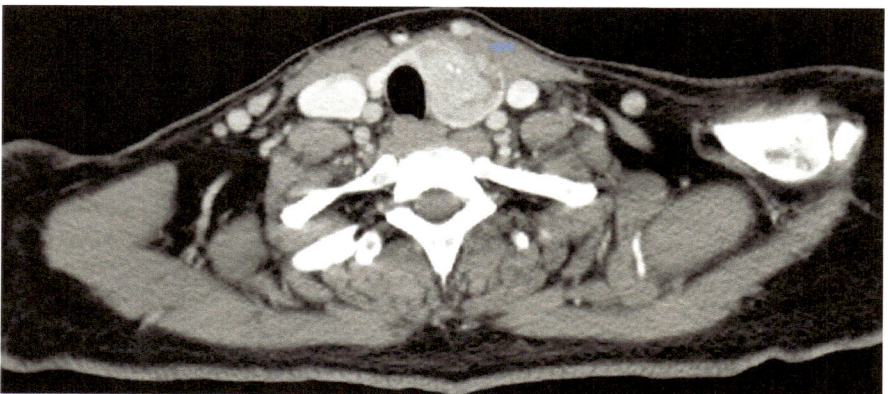

Fig. 7.8   Ca thyroid - notice the break in thyroid capsule

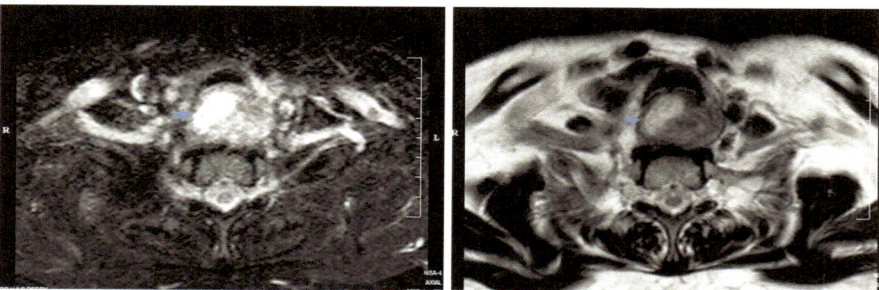

Fig. 7.9   Hurthle cell Ca axial MR (STIR and T1)

Fig. 7.10 (**a**) Ca thyroid involving right lobe. Note diffuse borders and local infiltration. (**b**) Ca thyroid coronal reconstruction of same patient

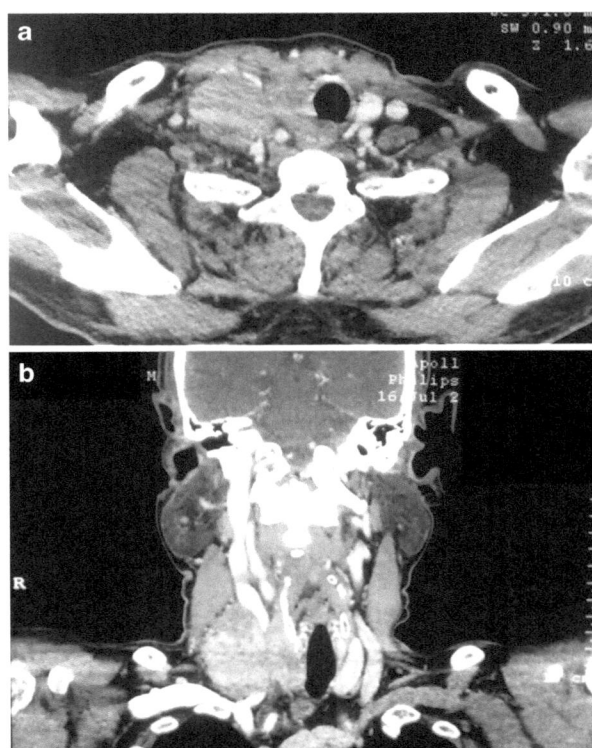

Fig. 7.11 (**a**) Ca thyroid
with tracheal infiltration.
(**b**) Ca thyroid coronal
reconstruction of same
patient

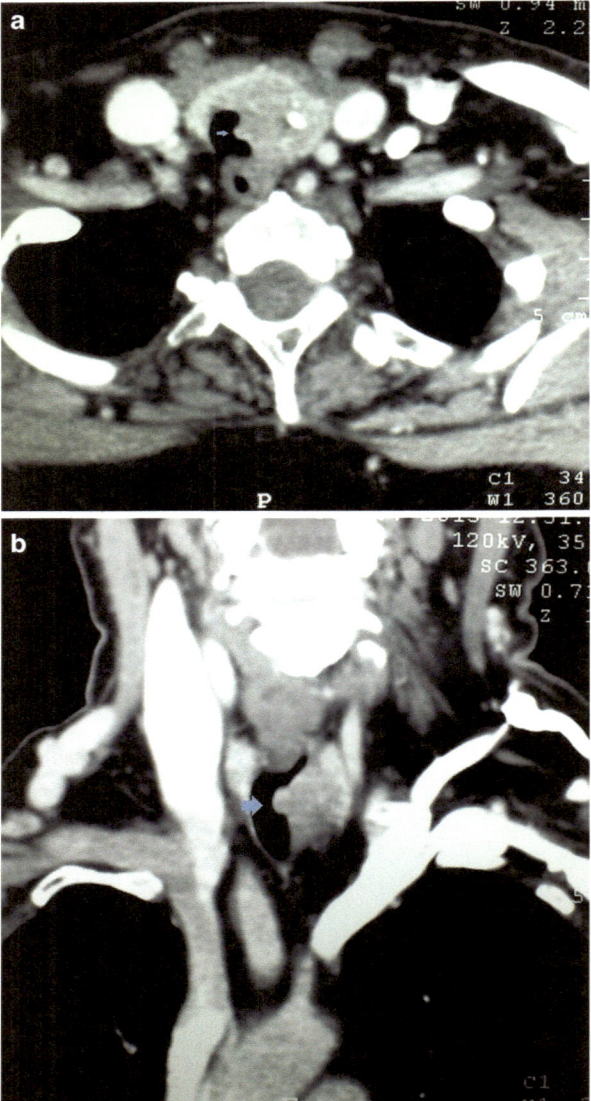

Fig. 7.12 Ca thyroid with
retrosternal extension

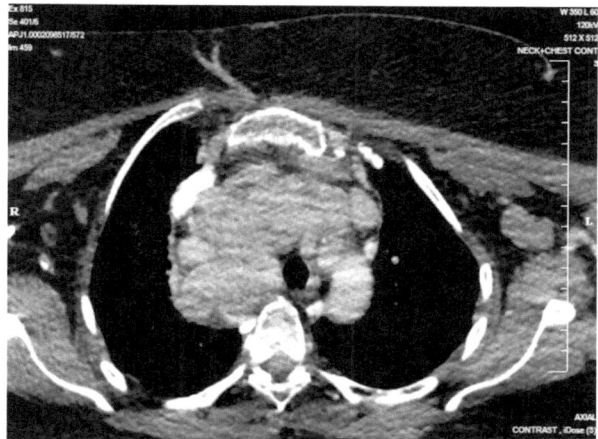

Fig. 7.13 Ca thyroid
post-thyroidectomy with
paratracheal recurrence

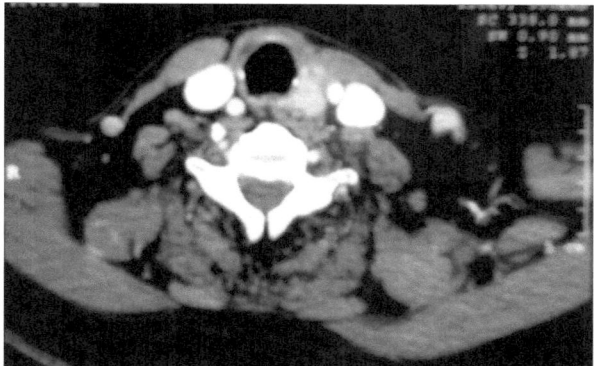

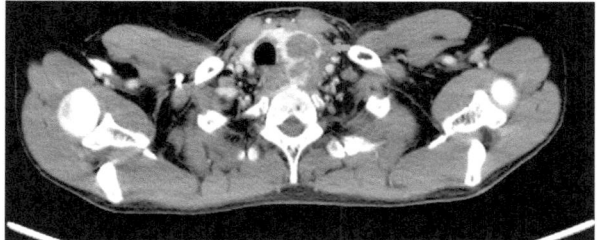

Fig. 7.14 Medullary Ca
thyroid

Fig. 7.15 Medullary Ca thyroid with mediastinal nodes

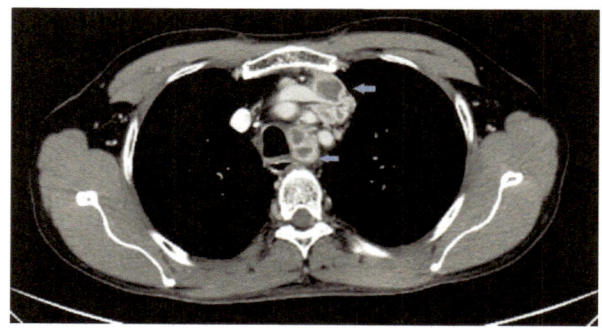

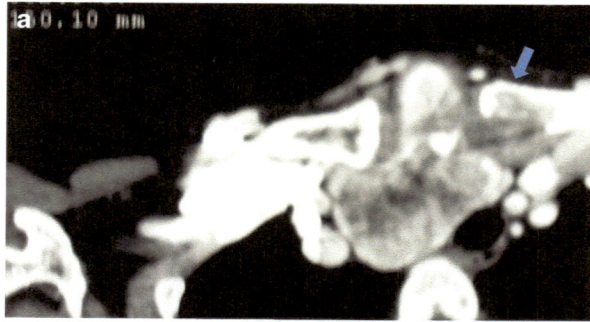

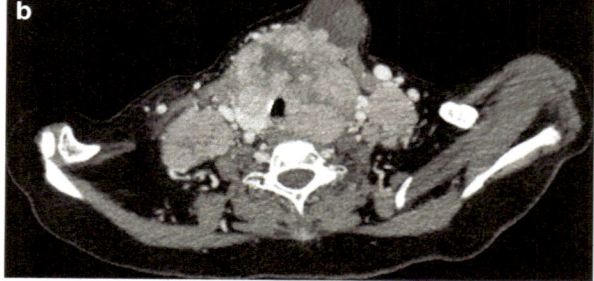

Fig. 7.16 (**a**) Ca thyroid with local infiltration into sternum and clavicle. (**b**) Anaplastic Ca thyroid with bilateral lymphadenopathy

Fig. 7.17 Non-Hodgkin's
lymphoma of thyroid

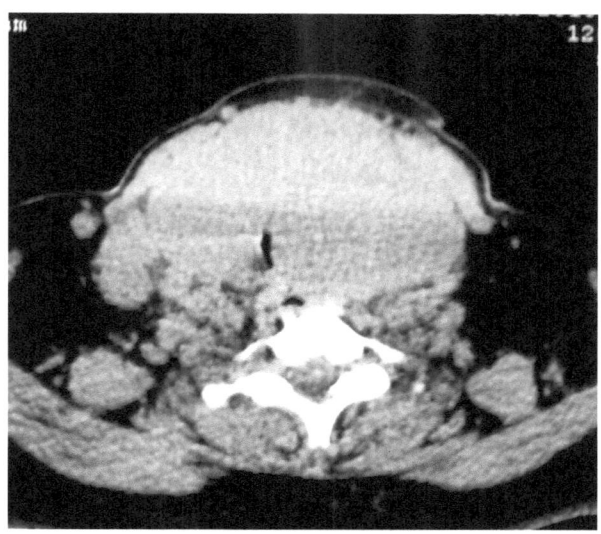

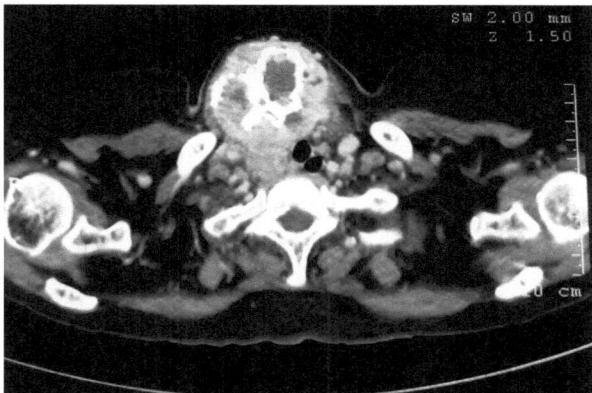

Fig. 7.18 Ca thyroid with
calcification axial CT
showing interrupted
egg-shell calcification

Fig. 7.19 Papillary Ca
thyroid with calcification
in long-standing right lobe
thyroid nodule

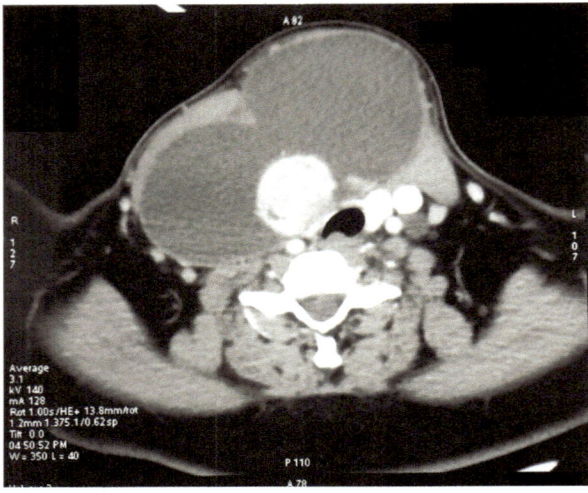

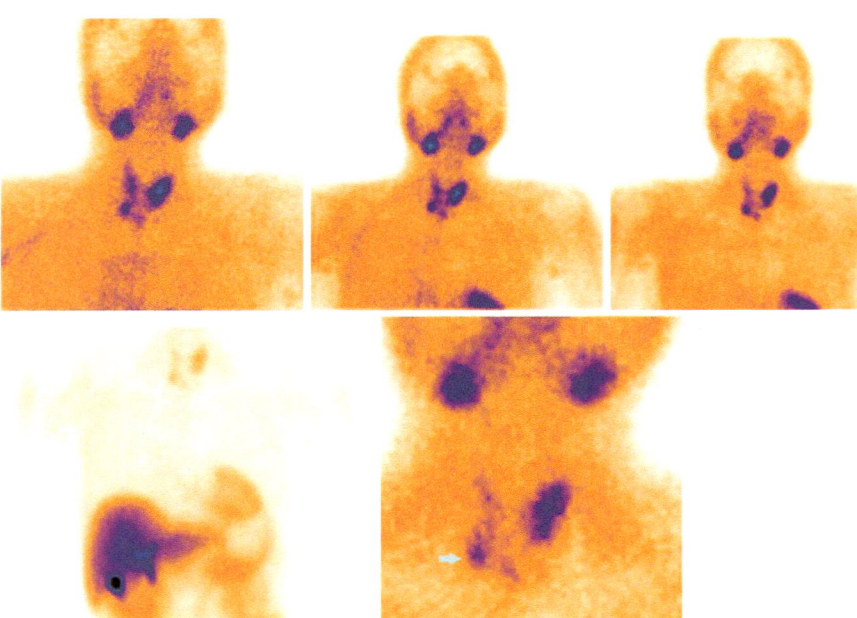

Fig. 7.20 Parathyroid adenoma sestamibi parathyroid scan

RT

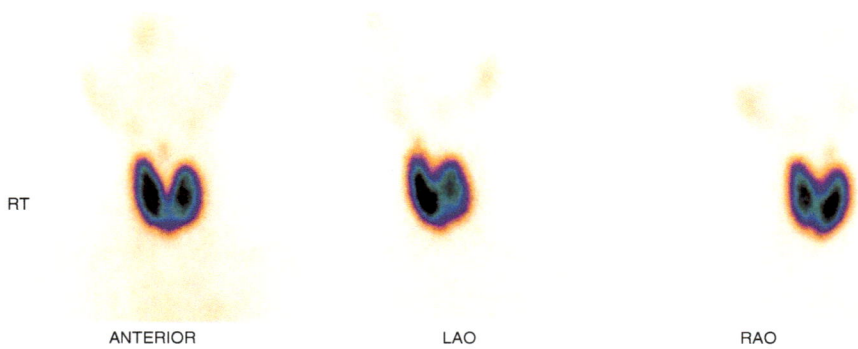

ANTERIOR   LAO   RAO

Fig. 7.21 Graves disease—technetium thyroid scan

Salivary Gland

Choice of Imaging

1. **MR** (fat suppressed) is generally preferred for the parotid gland since it delineates better extraparenchymal spread, deep lobe/parapharyngeal extension, and facial nerve involvement. It is also imaging of choice for recurrent tumors and minor salivary gland tumors of the oropharynx.
2. **CT** is the preferred modality for advanced parotid gland tumors extending to skull base or involving bone/vascular invasion and for minor salivary gland tumors involving the palate.
3. CT also scores over MR for evaluation of sialadenitis and can help identify and localize sialoliths with more accuracy.
4. Sialography is used for evaluation of the ductal pattern of salivary glands, to identify salivary calculi and rule out pathologies and neoplasms.

Early Stage Tumor

1. Imaging is necessary to
   (a) Rule out the presence of tumor in diffuse parotid enlargement to guide further workup (FNAC, etc)
   (b) Rule out deep lobe involvement
   (c) To help differentiate malignant from benign tumors—MR is preferred to assess local invasion
   (d) To determine the presence/absence of subclinical nodes in malignancies.
2. MR can aid in detecting perineural invasion in case of adenoid cystic Ca.
3. Imaging can also differentiate intraparotid nodes from primary parotid tumor.

© The Author(s) 2018
U. Nayak et al., *Clinical Radiology of Head and Neck Tumors*,
https://doi.org/10.1007/978-981-10-5036-7_8

Advanced Tumor

1. Imaging is mandatory in order to identify inoperability—skull base involvement, carotid artery infiltration, etc.
2. Deep lobe parotid tumor may be differentiated from a parapharyngeal tumor by the relative position of the parapharyngeal space fat displacement (medially in case of deep lobe tumors and laterally in parapharyngeal tumors).
3. Dumbbell-shaped tumor is seen when there is involvement of both superficial and deep lobe of the parotid.

Fig. 8.1 Pleomorphic
adenoma axial CT

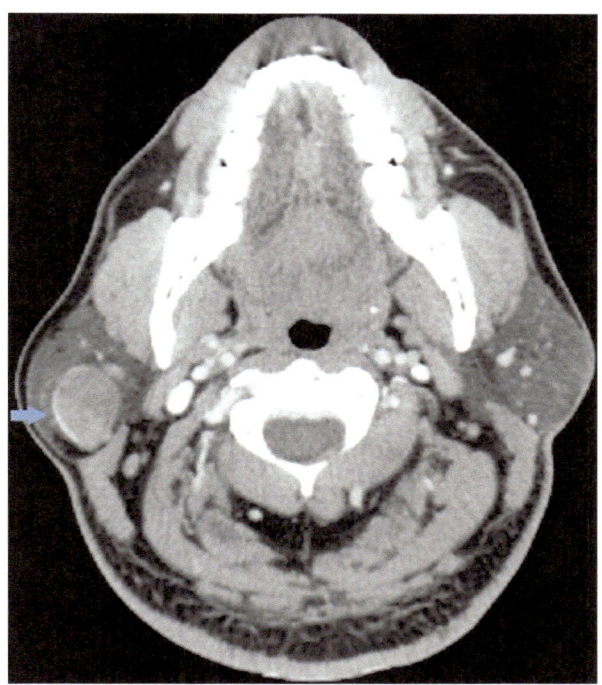

Fig. 8.2 Pleomorphic
adenoma deep lobe tumor
axial CT

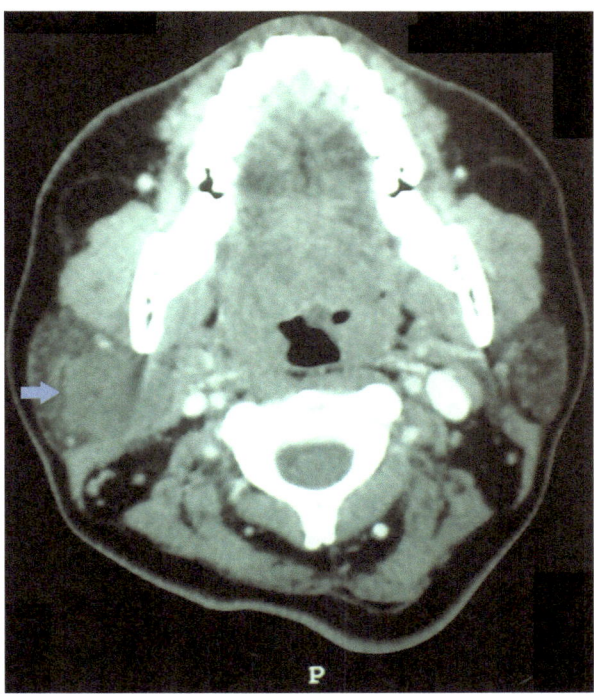

Fig. 8.3 Pleomorphic
Adenoma - Axial CT
showing large deep lobe
tumor mimicking
parapharyngeal tumor.
Note medial displacement
of parapharyngeal fat

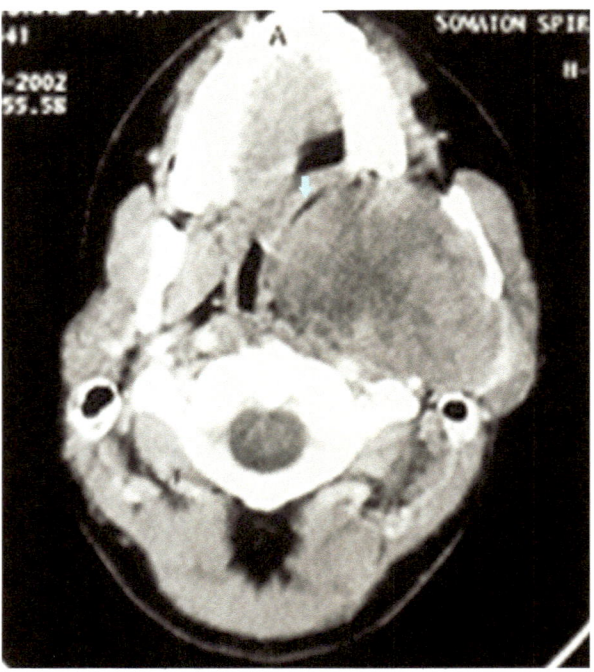

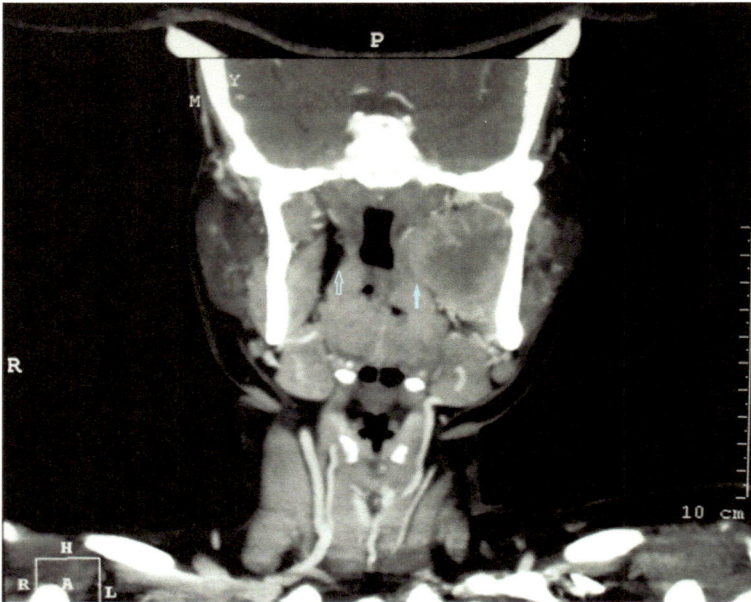

Fig. 8.4 Pleomorphic adenoma coronal CT showing left side deep lobe tumor. Normal parapharyngeal fat on *right* side and compressed fat on *left*

Fig. 8.5 Pleomorphic adenoma deep lobe MRI T1 contrast. Note again compression of parapharyngeal fat

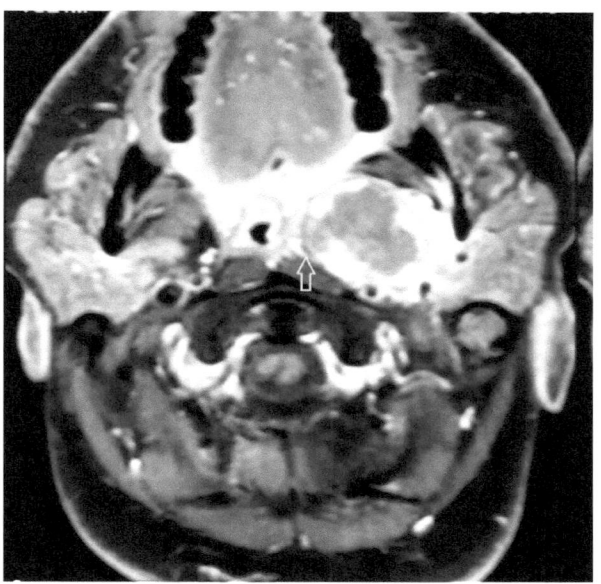

Fig. 8.6 (a) Dumbell
pleomorphic adenoma
involving superficial and
deep lobe axial CT.
(**b**) Dumbell pleomorphic
adenoma coronal CT of
same patient

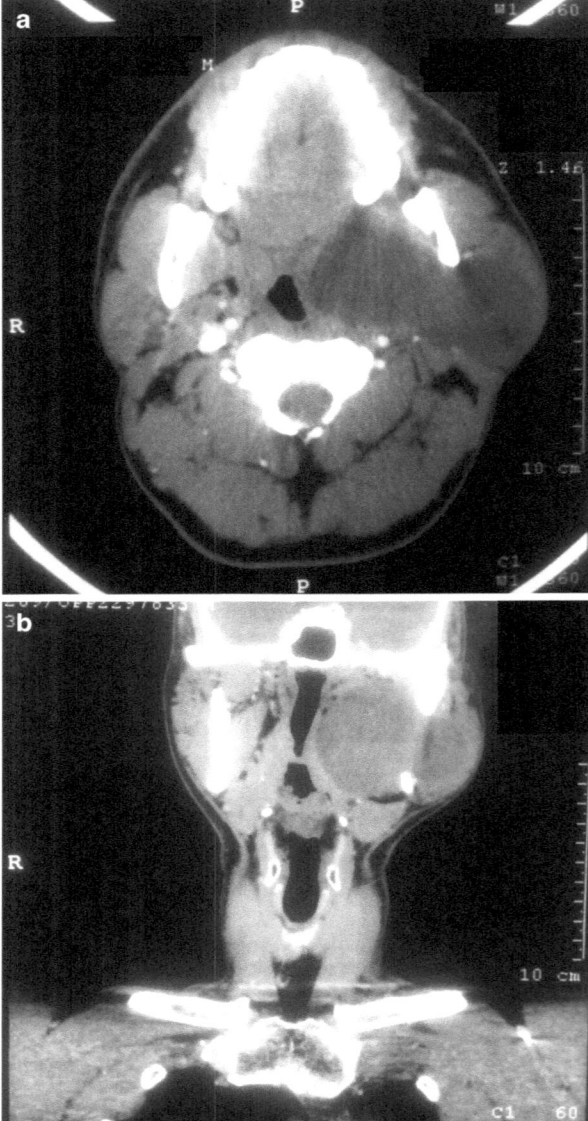

Fig. 8.7 (a) Warthin's tumor lower pole parotid axial CT. (b) Warthin's tumor lower pole—coronal CT of same patient clearly showing origin from parotid

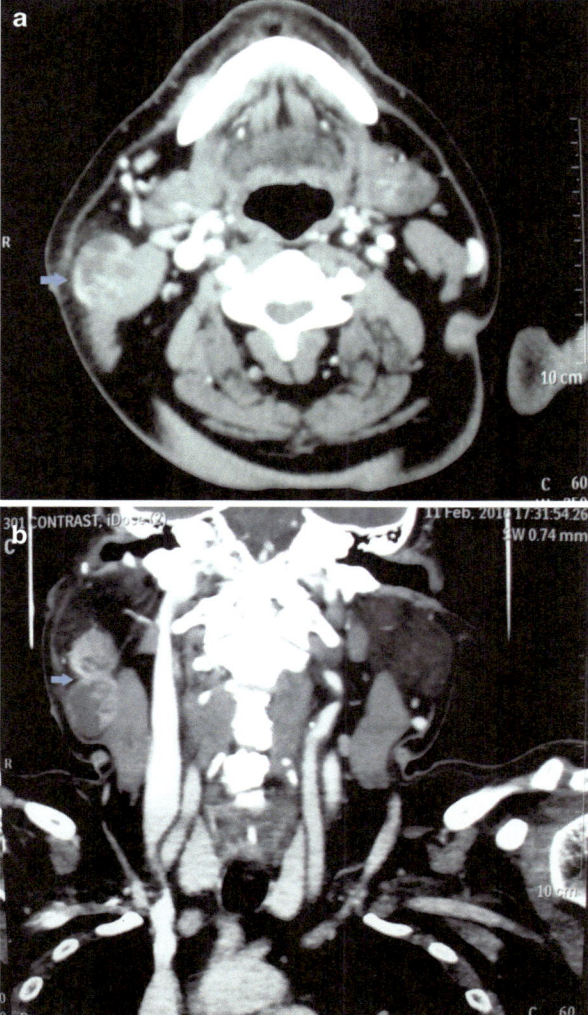

Fig. 8.8 Recurrent
pleomorphic adenoma
multicentric recurrence
deep lobe involving
infratemporal fossa

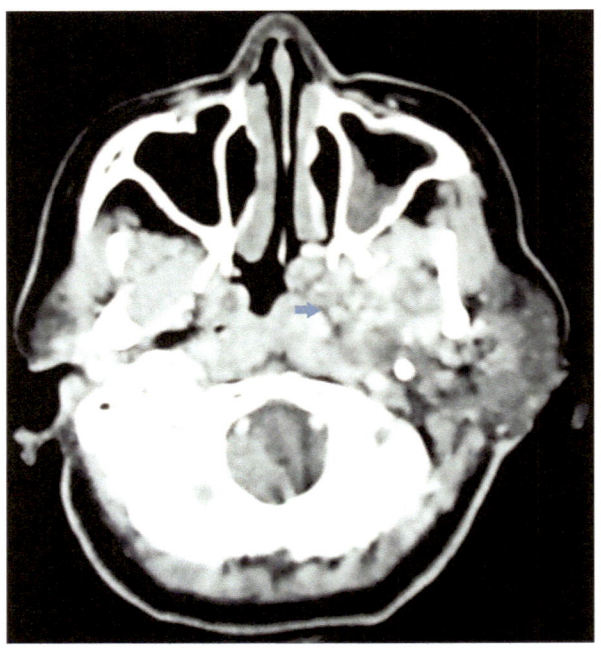

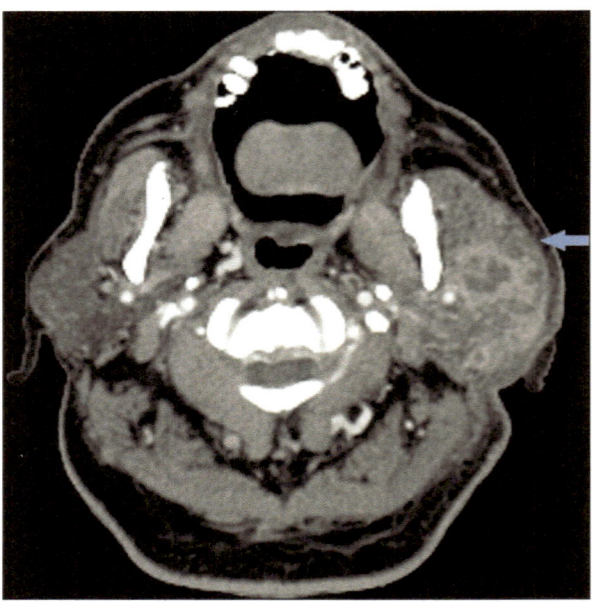

Fig. 8.9 Malignant left
parotid tumor axial CT

Fig. 8.10 Muco-epidermoid Ca coronal CT. Note irregular borders of tumor

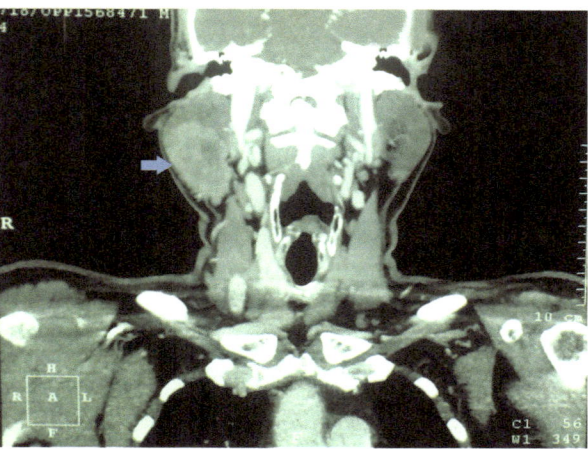

Fig. 8.11 (**a**) Muco-
epidermoid Ca parotid.
Axial CT showing tumor
closely related to facial
nerve area. (**b**) Muco-
epidermoid Ca parotid
Coronal reconstruction of
same patient. Intra-op
tumor was infiltrating
lower division of facial
nerve

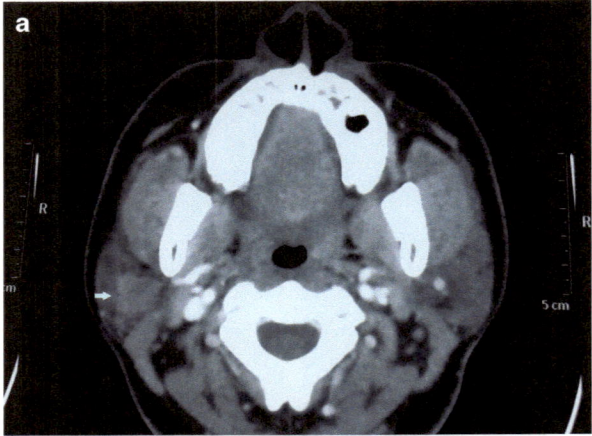

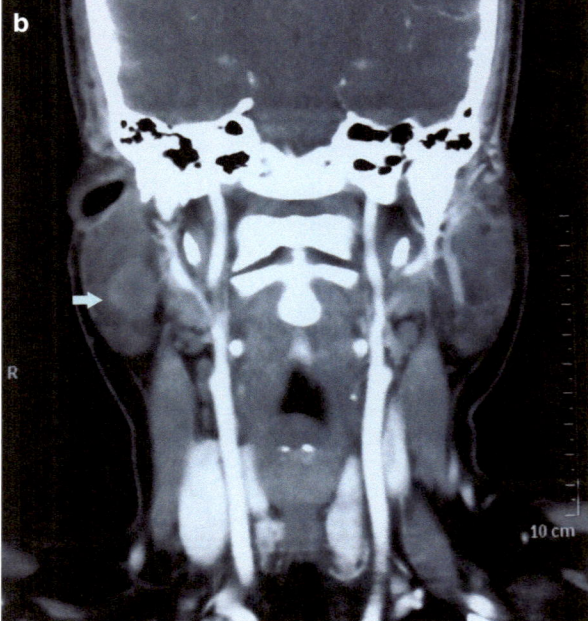

Fig. 8.12 Minor salivary gland tumor arising from hard palate showing resorption of bone axial CT

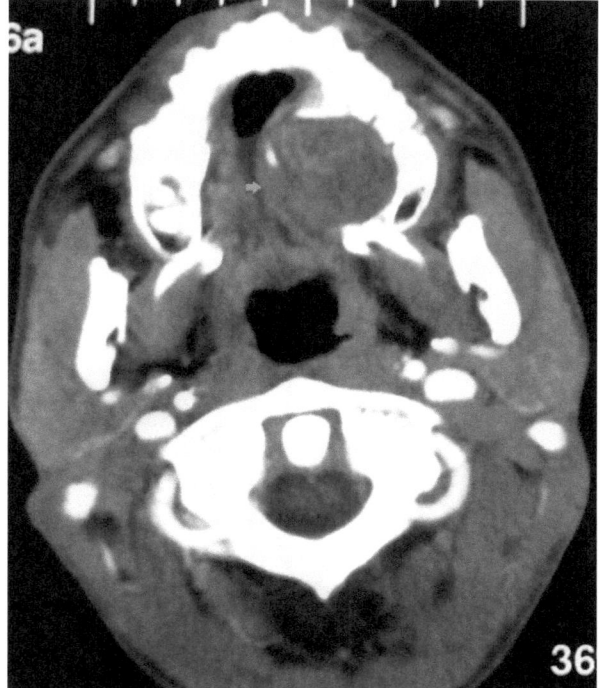

Fig. 8.13 (**a**) Minor
salivary gland tumor
infratemporal fossa axial
CT. (**b**) Minor salivary
gland tumor infratemporal
fossa—coronal
reconstruction of same
patient showing tumor
extension upto base of
skull

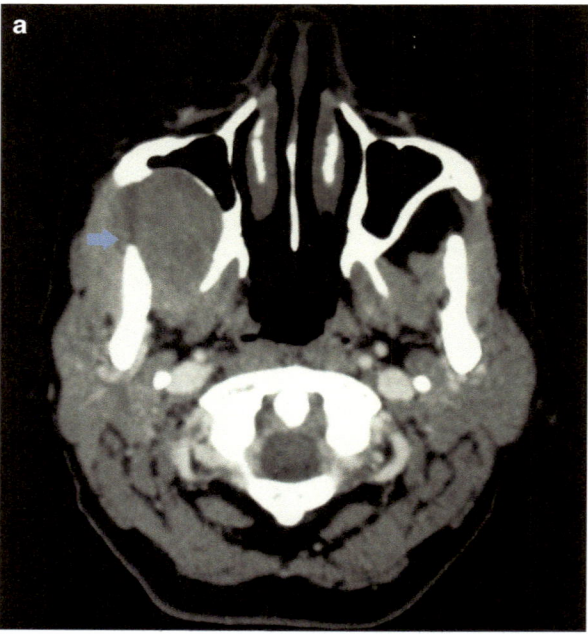

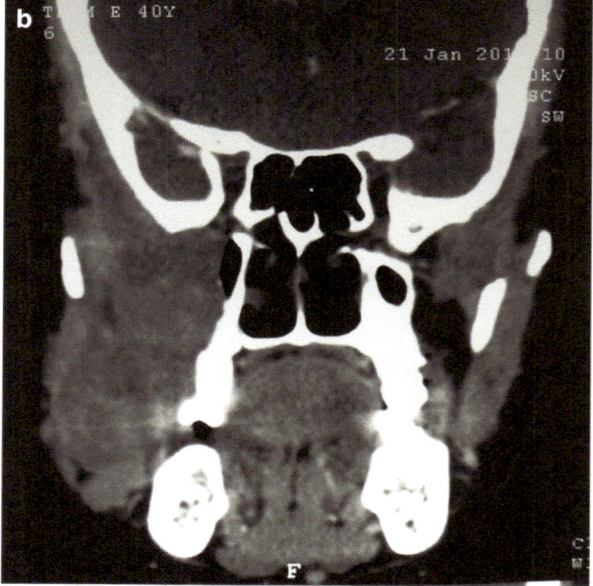

Fig. 8.14 (**a**) Parotitis axial CT demonstrating calculi. (**b**) Parotitis with calculi—coronal reconstruction

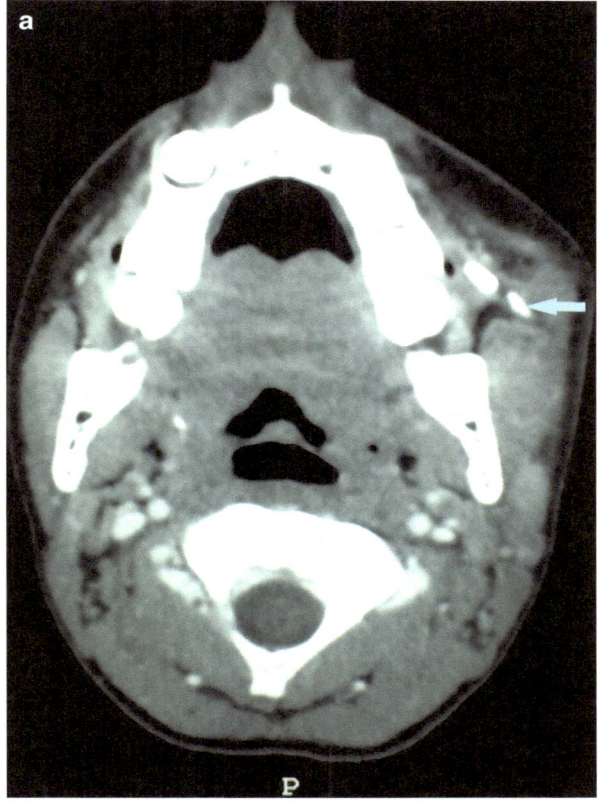

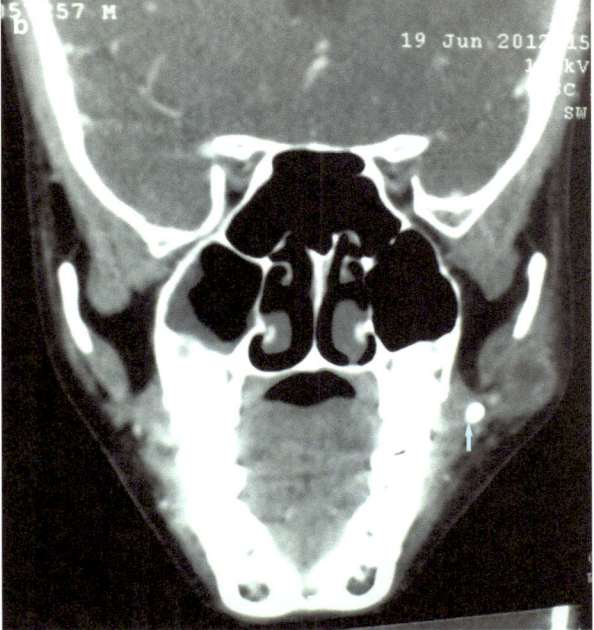

Fig. 8.15 Ranula
extending to involve
submandibular gland

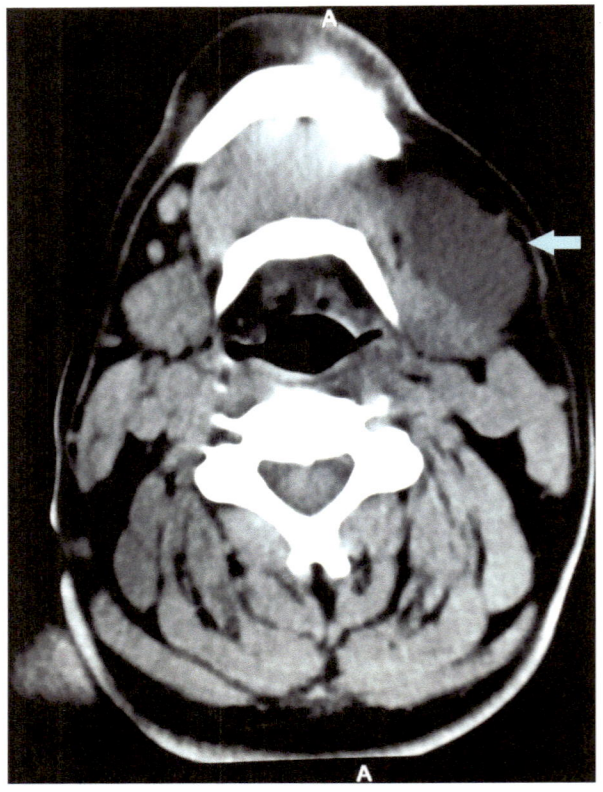

Choice of Imaging

1. **MR** is generally preferred since it shows mucosal and parapharyngeal extensions better while CT is reserved for cases with skull base and spine involvement.
2. **CT** is the imaging of choice for nasopharyngeal angiofibromas in view of their vascularity but once they extend intracranially, MR provides better idea of the extensions.
3. **Angiography** and preoperative embolization is generally preferred in cases of angiofibromas prior to surgical excision.
4. **PET-CT** is the imaging modality of choice for assessing post treatment relapses in Ca nasopharynx as well as in evaluation of lymphomas involving the nasopharynx.
5. In MUO (metastasis of unknown origin), CT or PET-CT may help identification of occult primary in nasopharynx.

© The Author(s) 2018
U. Nayak et al., *Clinical Radiology of Head and Neck Tumors*,
https://doi.org/10.1007/978-981-10-5036-7_9

Fig. 9.1 (**a**) Nasopharyngeal angiofibroma CT axial showing tumor extending into pterygo-palatine fossa. (**b**) Coronal reconstruction of same patient showing erosion of greater sphenoid wing

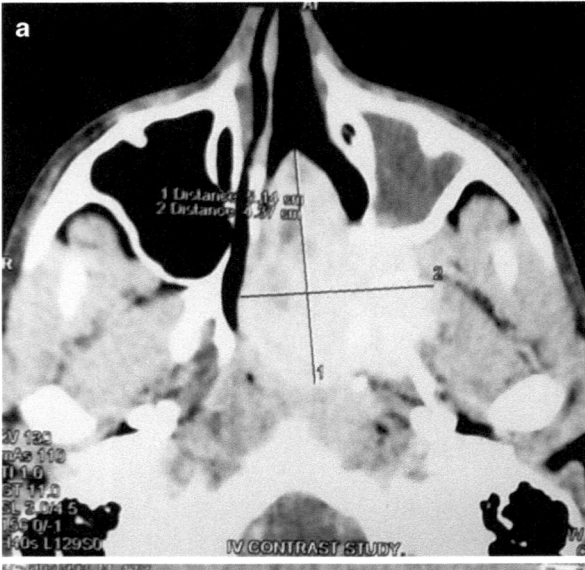

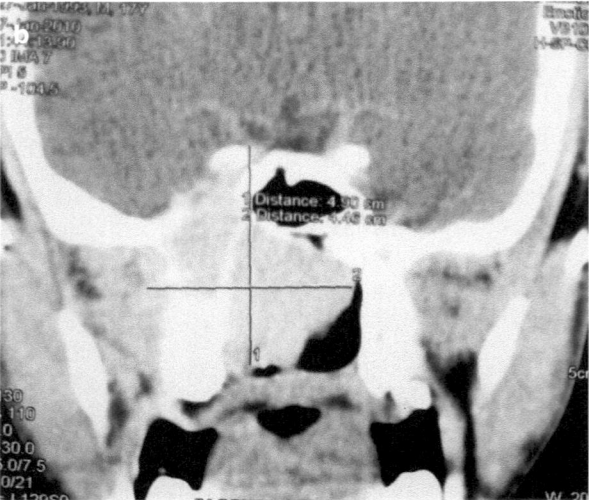

Fig. 9.2 Nasopharyngeal angiofibroma extending to sphenoid sinus and infratemporal fossa-coronal reconstruction

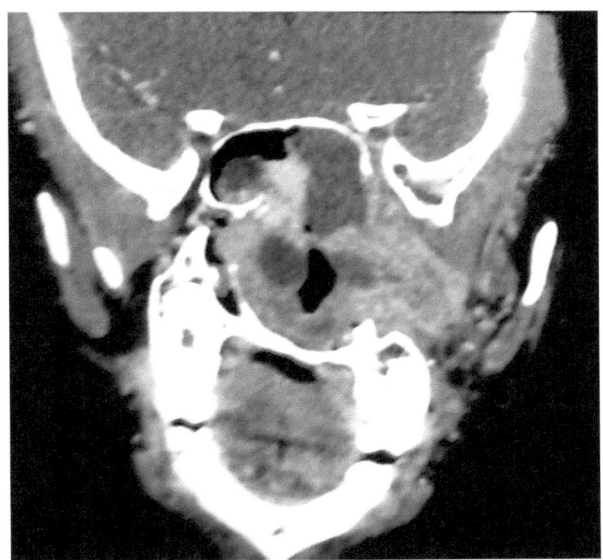

Fig. 9.3 (**a**) Angiofibroma with intracranial extension coronal CT. (**b**) Coronal MRI T1 sequence of same patient giving better idea of tumor extensions

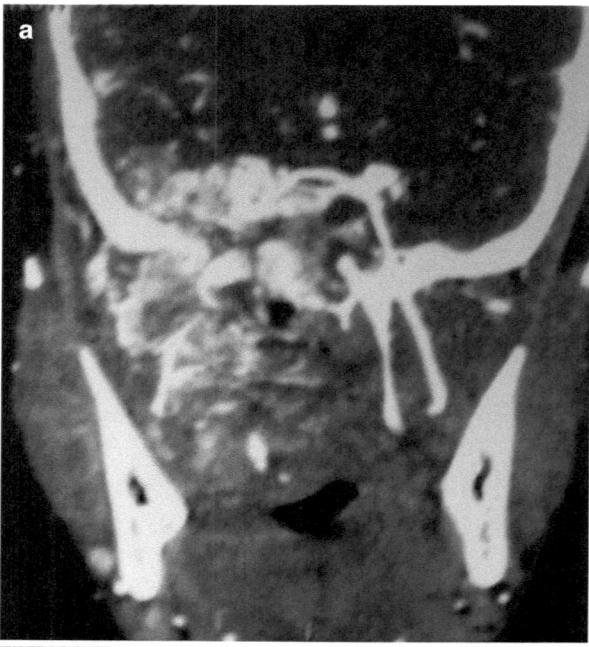

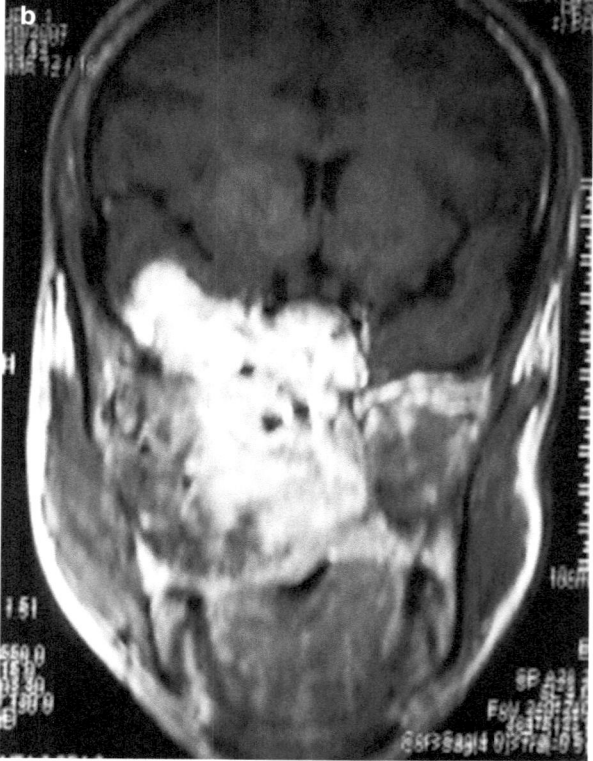

Fig. 9.4 (**a**) Ca nasopharynx CT axial showing nasopharyngeal mass suggestive of Ca nasopharynx. (**b**) Ca nasopharynx lower axial CT sections of same patient showing large metastatic node in upper posterior triangle

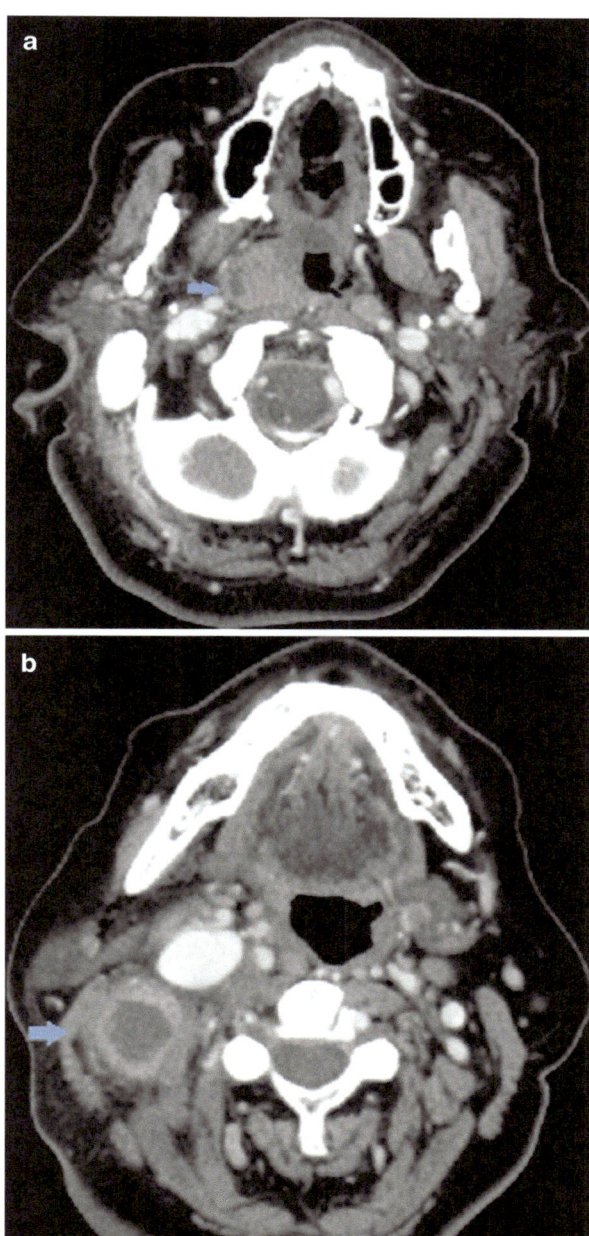

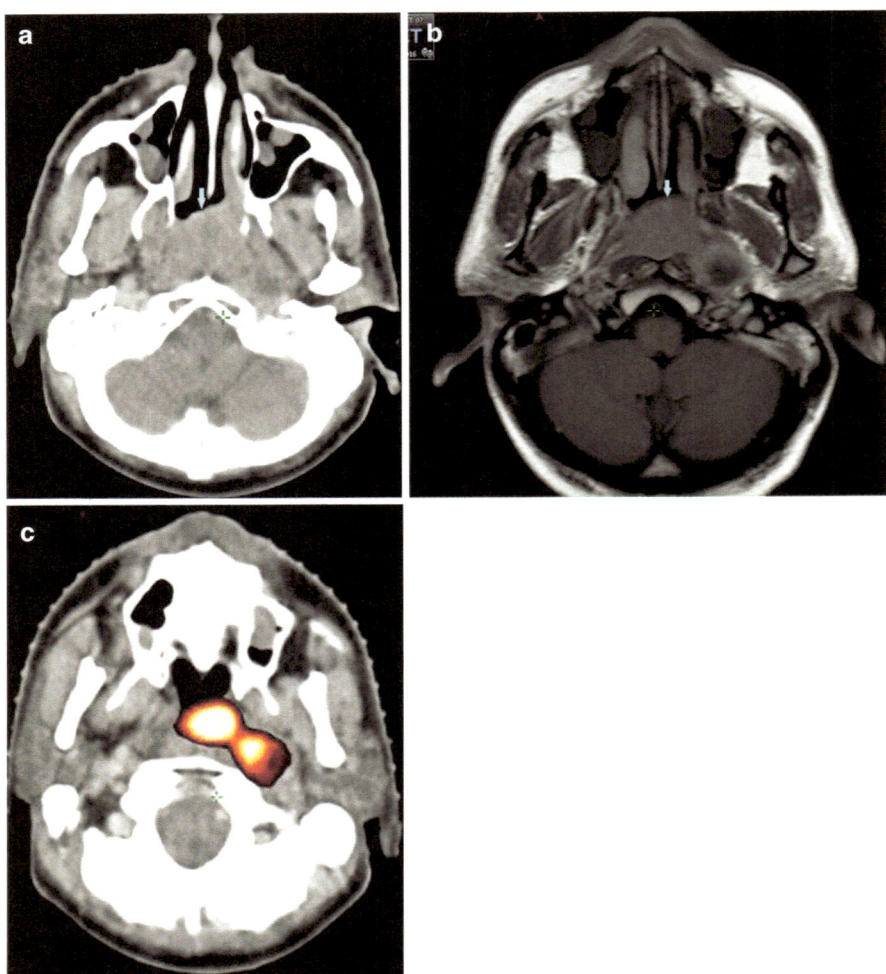

Fig. 9.5 (**a**) Ca nasopharynx T3 axial CT. (**b**) Ca nasopharynx T1 axial MR of same patient. (**c**) Ca nasopharynx PET CT (same patient)

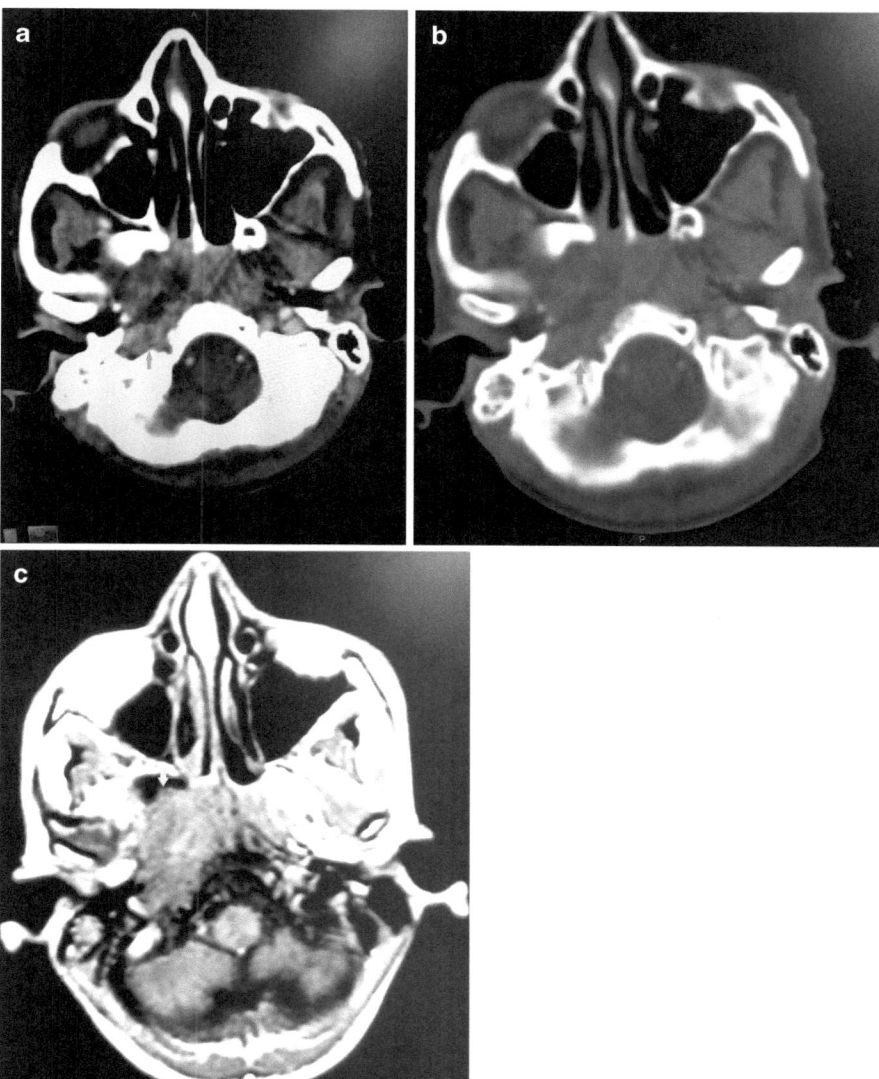

Fig. 9.6 (**a**) Ca nasopharynx T4 with skull base erosion axial CT. (**b**) Ca nasopharynx T4 with skull base erosion bone window. (**c**) Ca nasopharynx same patient-axial MR

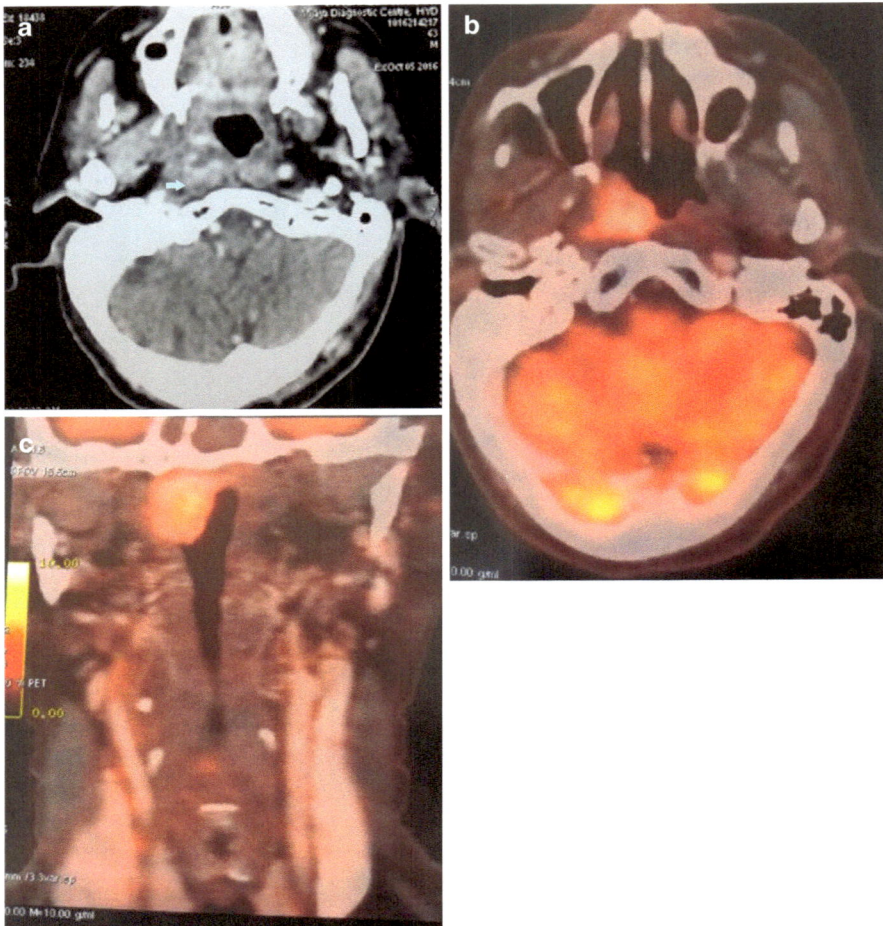

Fig. 9.7 (**a**) Post CT RT relapse Ca nasopharynx. (**b**) Ca nasopharynx post CTRT axial PET-CT. (**c**) Ca nasopharynx post CTRT coronal PET-CT

Proper imaging in the form of CT and/or MR is mandatory in evaluation of all PNS and skull base tumors since clinical evaluation gives limited information regarding extent, nature, and operability. Because of the rarity and wide range of some of these tumors as well as difficulties in obtaining a biopsy due to their deep location within the facial skeleton, imaging plays a vital role in their diagnosis and management.

Choice of Imaging

Paranasal Sinus and Orbit

1. **CT** is generally the imaging modality of choice in view of the bony configuration of the paranasal sinus.
2. **MR** helps differentiate between tumor and mucosal thickening/retained secretions caused by obstruction to the sinus opening as well as for problem-solving, where CT fails to give a clear picture. It is also preferred for lesions which have breached the skull base to assess dura and brain involvement.
3. In the orbit CT aids in detecting breach of orbital walls but MR can better demonstrate involvement of periorbita, orbital fat, and orbital apex which can influence surgical management.

© The Author(s) 2018
U. Nayak et al., *Clinical Radiology of Head and Neck Tumors*,
https://doi.org/10.1007/978-981-10-5036-7_10

Skull Base

1. Both CT and MR complement each other for skull base lesions with CT indicating breach of anterior or middle cranial fossa mandating craniofacial resection and MR demonstrating involvement of brain parenchyma and cavernous sinus indicating inoperability.
2. Dural and perineural invasion are also better assessed by MR.
3. Encirclement of internal carotid artery by tumor requires MR or CT angiography, generally more than 270° encirclement of ICA is an indication for carotid artery resection. Conventional angiography with balloon test occlusion is to be performed in case resection of ICA is contemplated in order to assess flow from contralateral ICA through Circle of Willis.

Fig. 10.1 Ossifying
fibroma ethmoid - CT plain
axial showing tumor
pushing into orbit

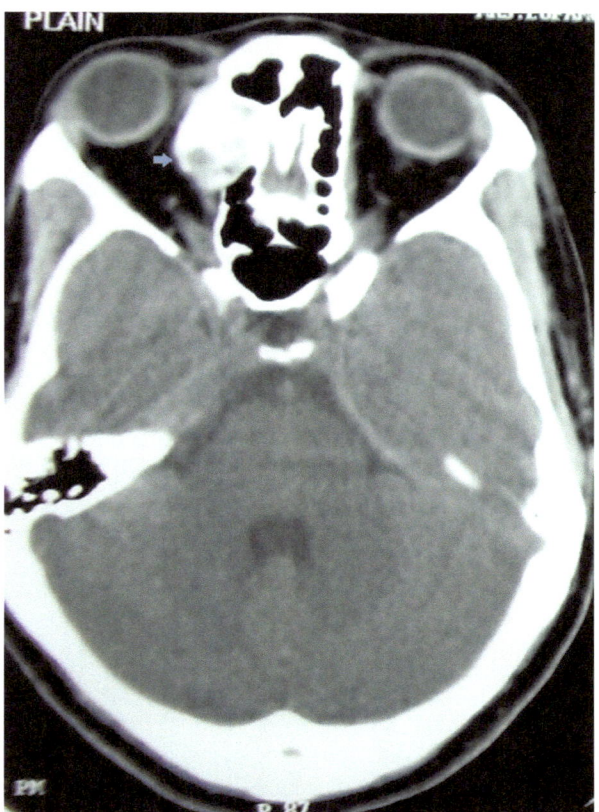

Fig. 10.2 Large ossifying
fibroma maxilla coronal
reconstruction

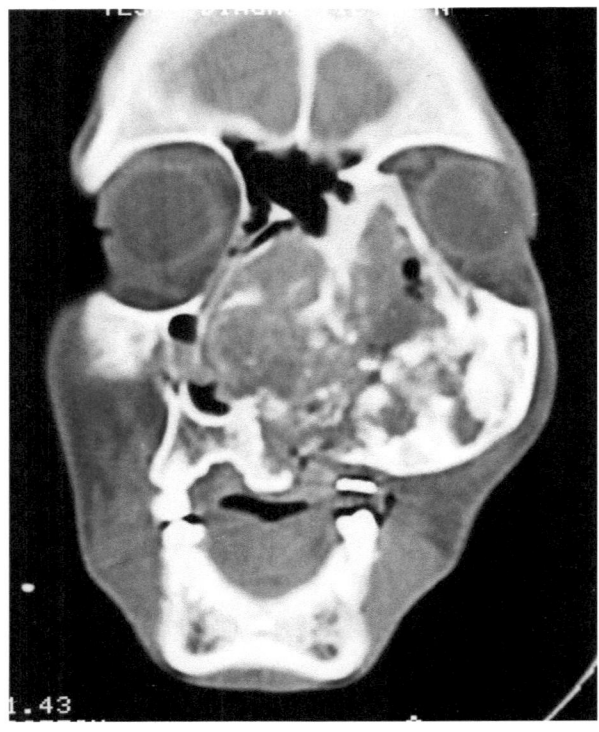

Fig. 10.3 Pleomorphic adenoma maxillary sinus (**a**) Axial CT showing tumor obliterating left maxillary sinus and eroding posterior wall (**b**) Coronal reconstruction of same patient showing intact skull base

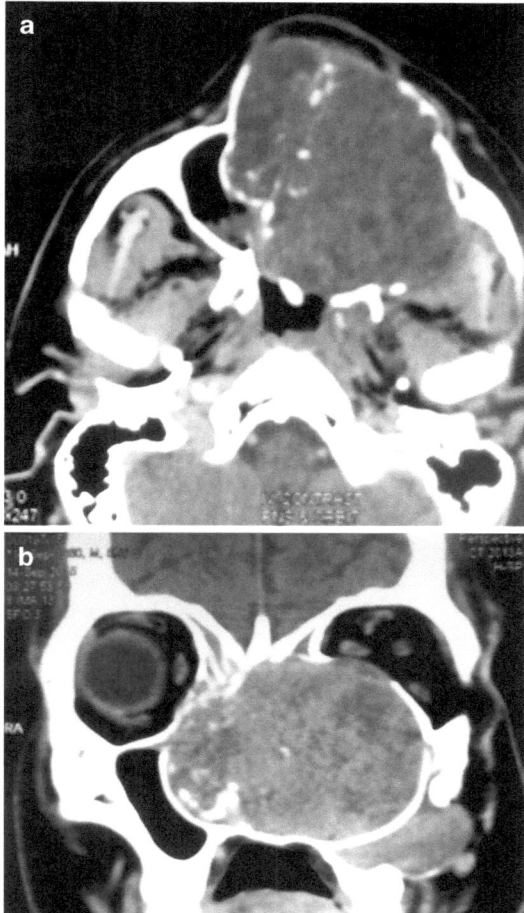

Fig. 10.4 (**a**) Ca maxillary
sinus coronal
reconstruction showing
tumor extending into oral
cavity. (**b**) Sagittal image
of same patient
demonstrating intact
orbital floor

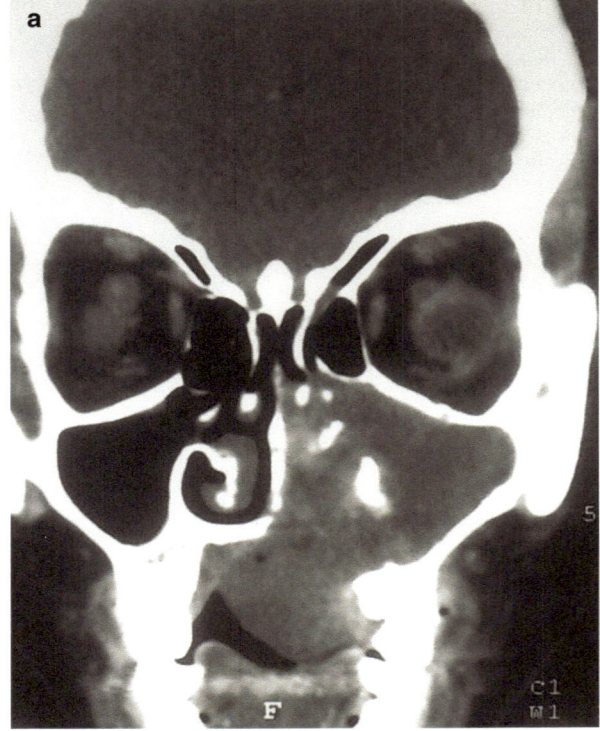

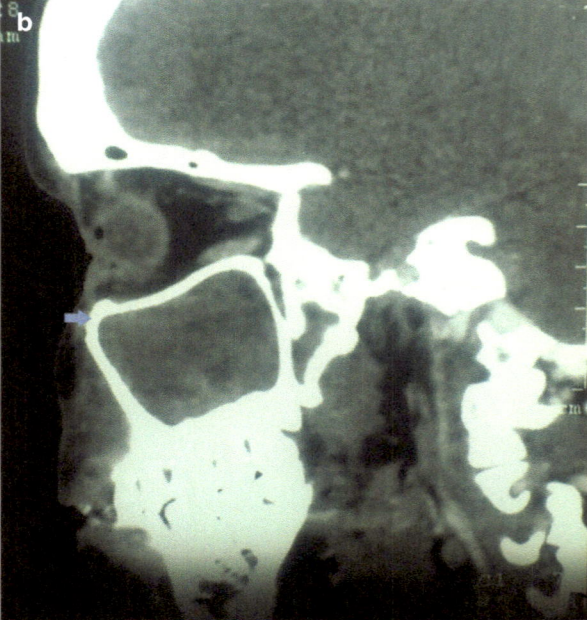

Fig. 10.5 Ca maxillary sinus coronal reconstruction demonstrating tumor invading floor of middle cranial fossa

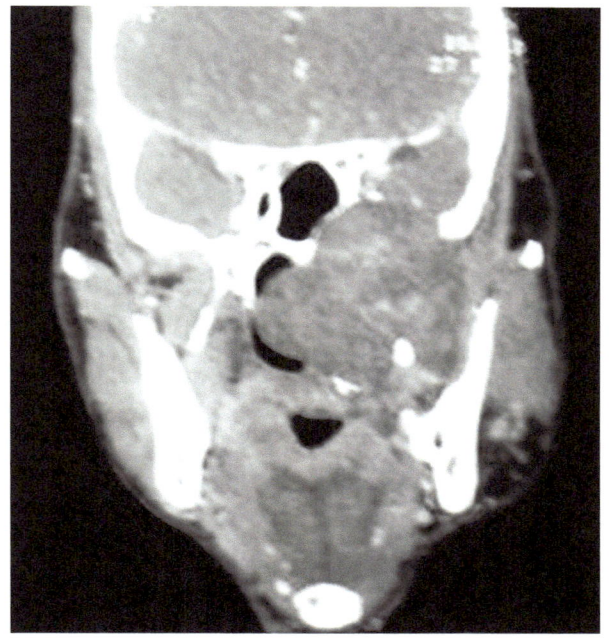

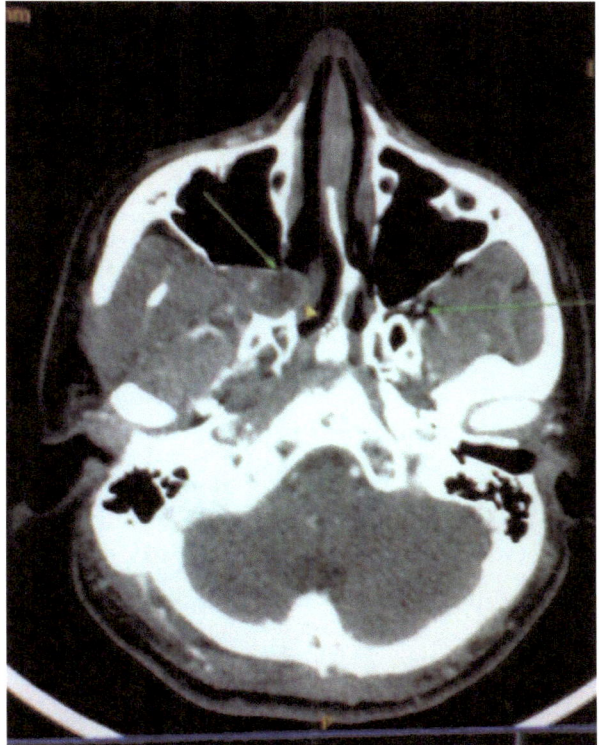

Fig. 10.6 Adenoid cystic Ca infratemporal fossa. Axial CT demonstrating widened pterygo-maxillary fissure on the right side, normal fissure on left

Fig. 10.7
(**a**) Infratemporal fossa
tumor CT axial.
(**b**) Coronal reconstruction
of same patient

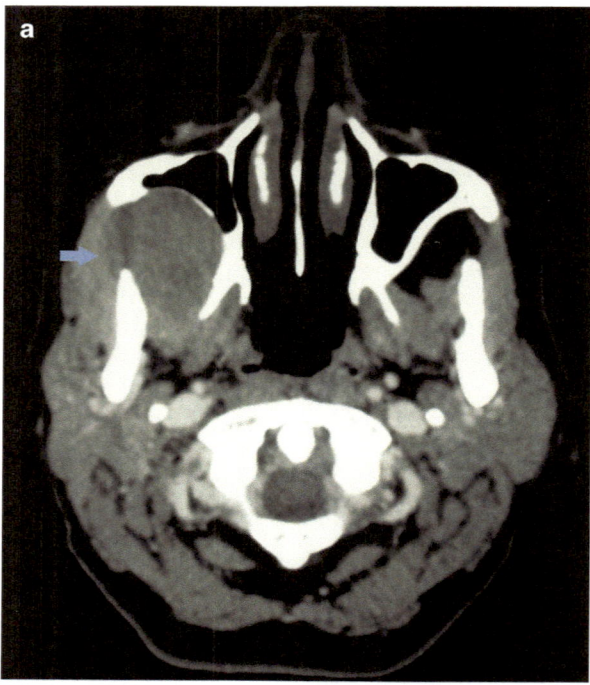

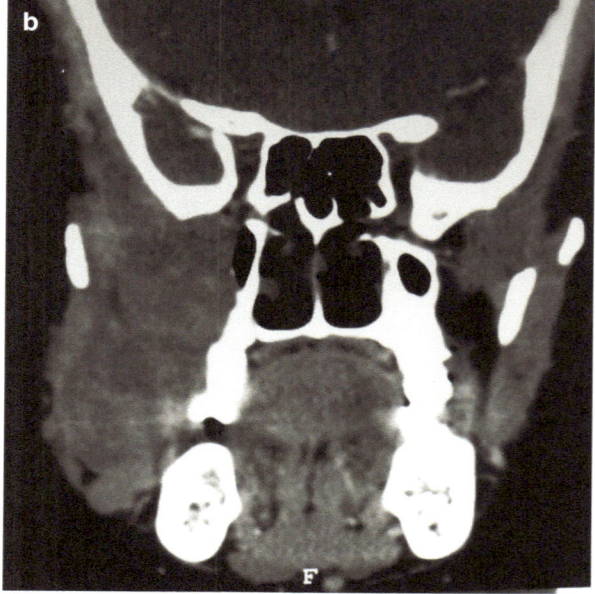

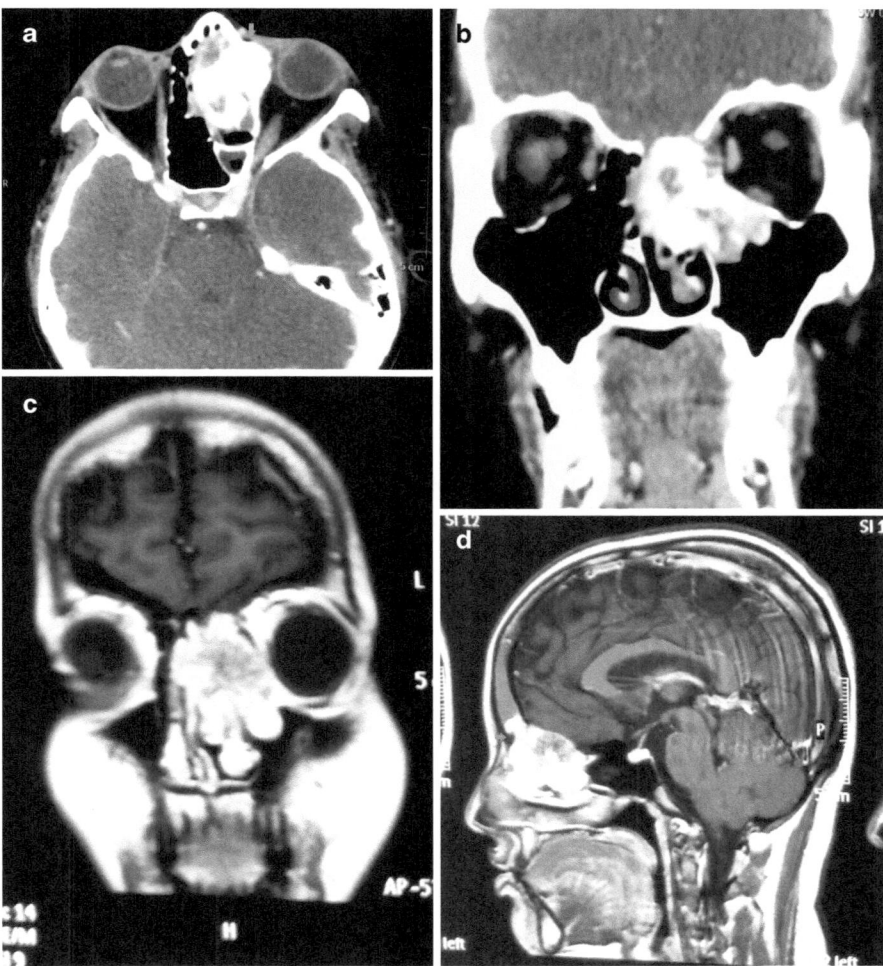

Fig. 10.8 (**a**) Osteosarcoma anterior skull base axial CT. (**b**) Coronal reconstruction demonstrating erosion af anterior skull base. (**c**) Osteosarcoma anterior skull base coronal MRI (same patient). (**d**) Sagittal MR of same patient showing intact dura and tumor has not breached through it

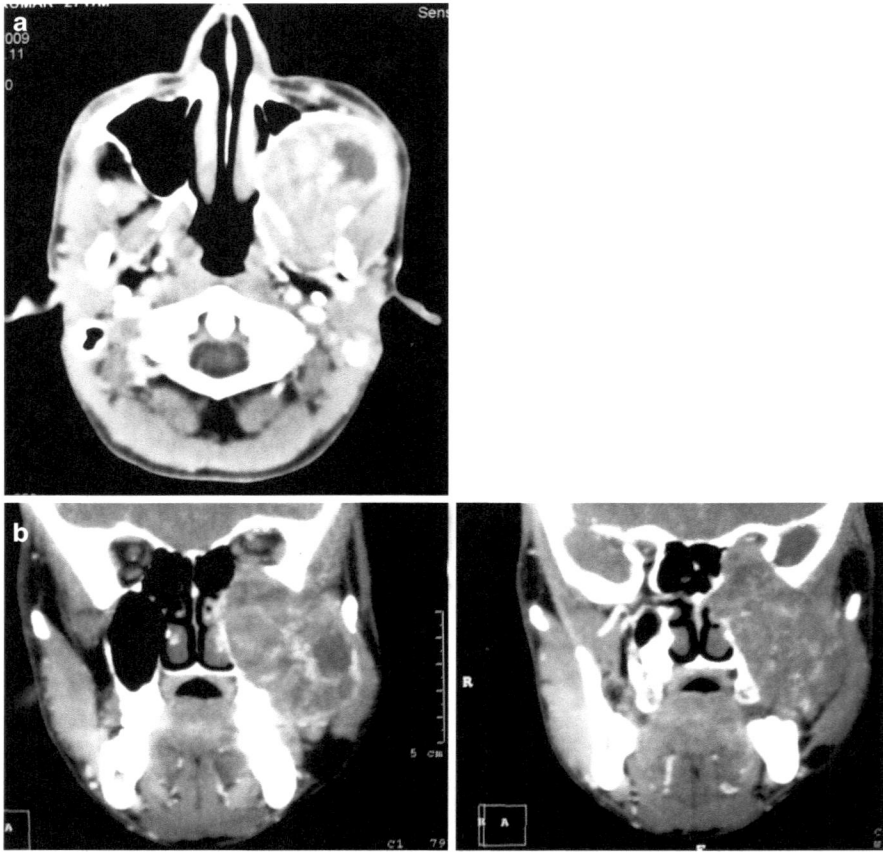

Fig. 10.9 (a) Skull base schwannoma axial CT. (b) Coronal CT of same patient demonstrating tumor getting into orbit and sphenoid sinus

Fig. 10.10 Skull base neurofibroma coronal reconstruction showing skull base erosion due to long-standing tumor

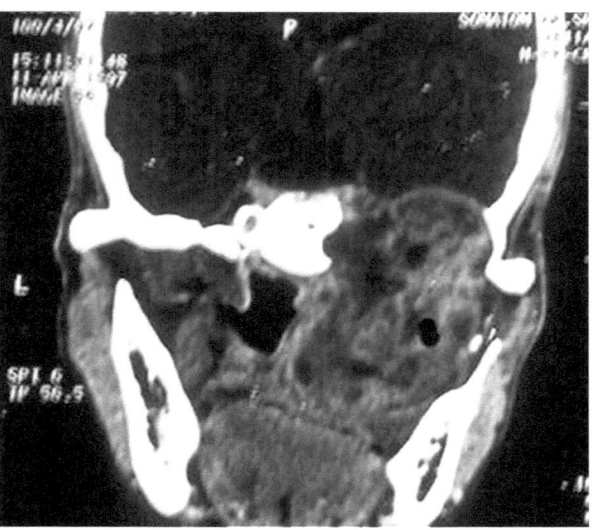

Fig. 10.11 (**a**) Spindle cell sarcoma skull base. Coronal CT (bone window) of a 2-year child demonstrating erosion of greater wing of sphenoid.(**b**) Coronal MR (T1) of same patient. Dura probably involved, brain not involved.

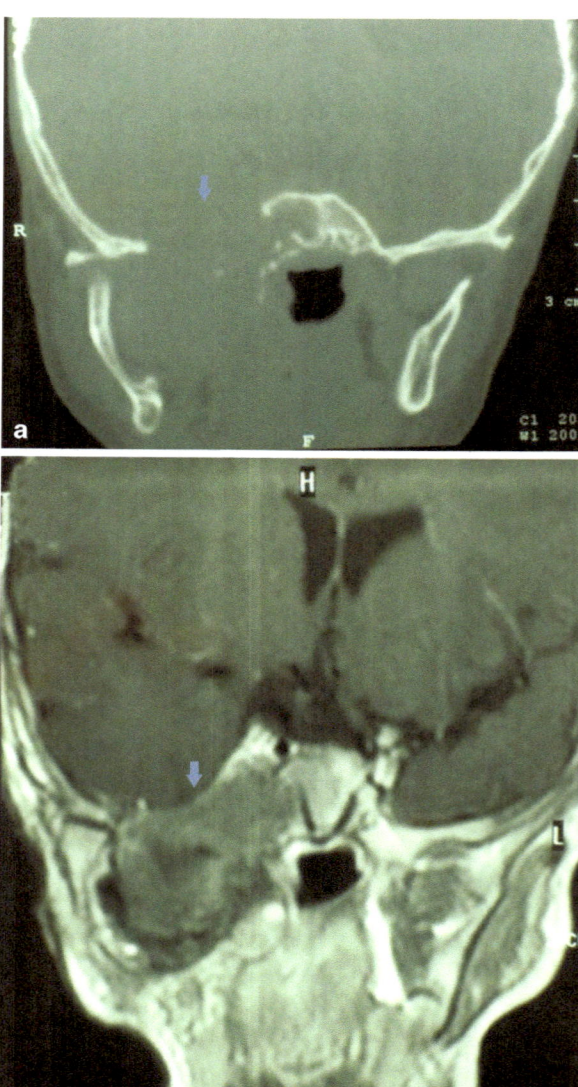

Fig. 10.12 Skull base malignant tumor with brain invasion axial MR showing tumor invading orbit and brain

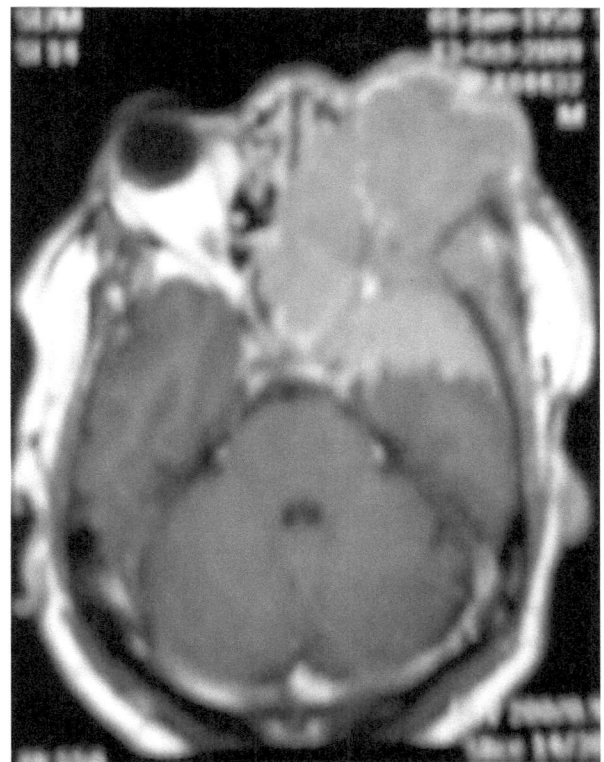

Fig. 10.13 Malignant
schwannoma MR T1
showing skull base erosion,
dural invasion and tumor
extension into cavernous
sinus

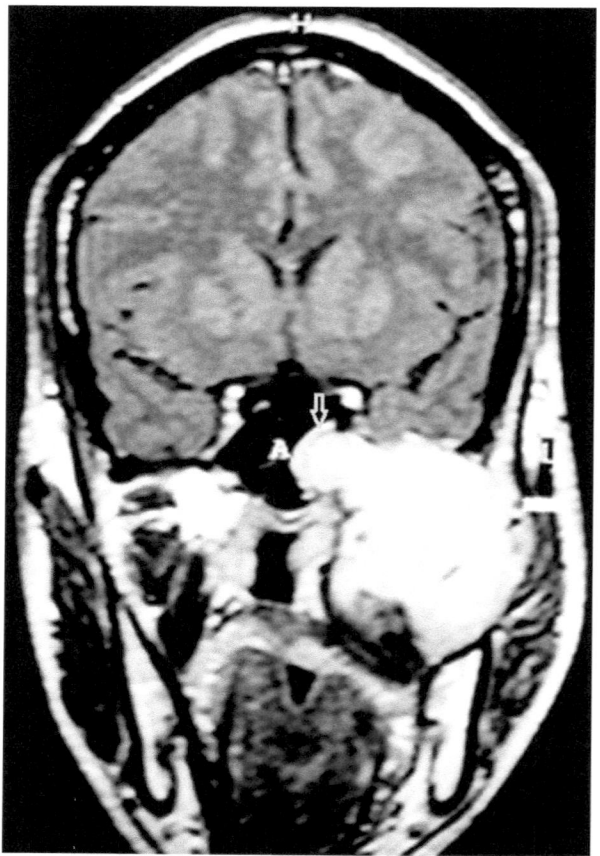

Fig. 10.14 Meningocoele -
Herniation of meningeal
contents into nasal cavity
through skull base defect
following surgery

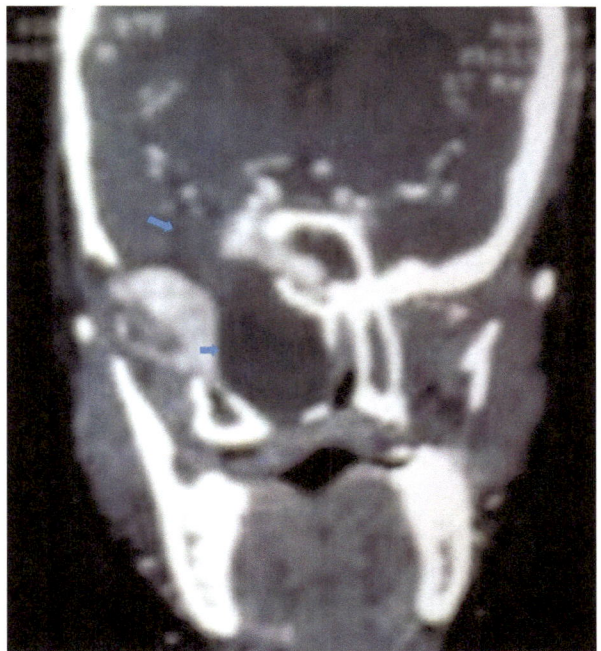

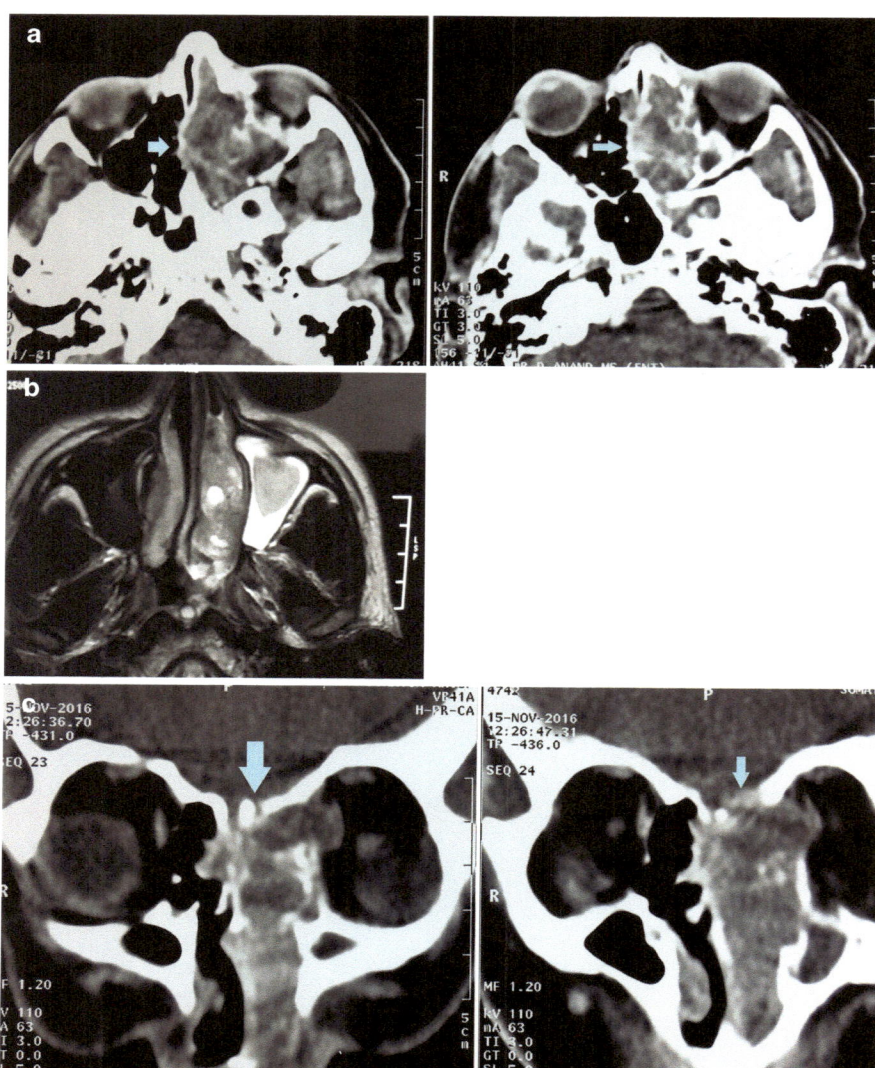

Fig. 10.15 (**a**) Inverted papilloma with squamous cell Ca differentiation. Axial CT. (**b**) Axial MR T1 contrast (same patient) left maxillary sinus showing retained secretions. (**c**) Inverted papilloma with squamous cell Ca differentiation. Coronal CT of same patient demonstrating erosion of cribriform plate. (**d**) Inverted papilloma with squamous cell Ca differentiation. Bone window. (**e**) Coronal MR T2 of same patient, left maxillary sinus showing retained secretions

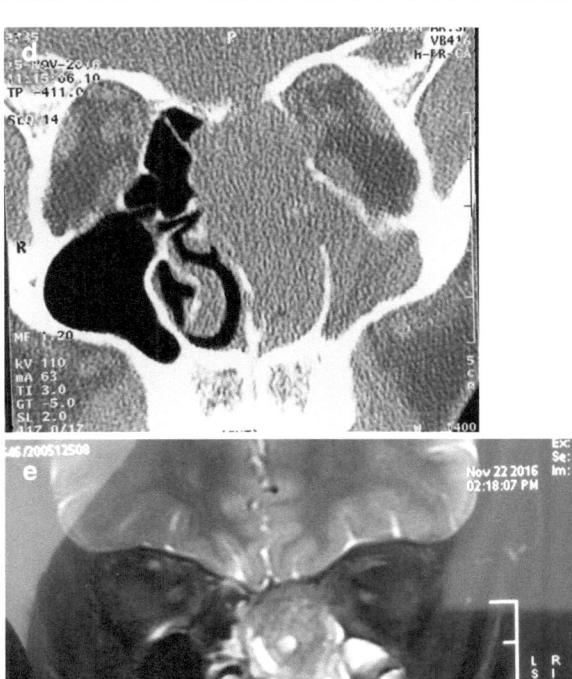

Fig. 10.15 (continued)

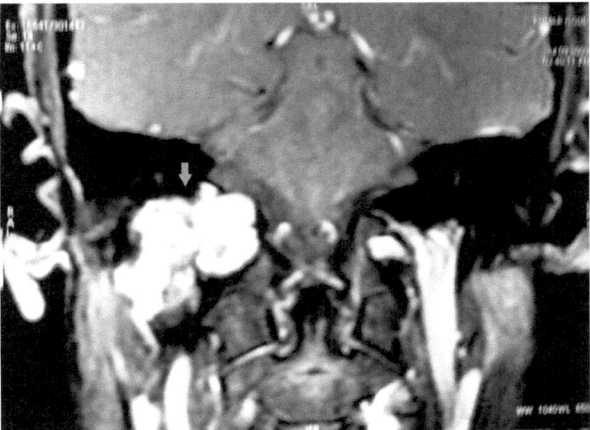

Fig. 10.16 Paraganglioma jugular foramen coronal MR T1 contrast

Vascular Tumors

Though comparatively rare, management of these tumors is challenging. Accurate imaging and diagnosis aids in reducing morbidity of surgery and helps counsel patients regarding possible risks.

Choice of Imaging

1. **USG with Doppler, CT, or MR** may be used in the initial evaluation of vascular tumors of head and neck. CT gives superior resolution of the vessels and defines tumor characteristics better. Coronal reconstruction provides the longitudinal extent of the tumor, skull base extension as well as relationship to the vessels and the vagus nerve while axial images assess the degree of encirclement of carotid artery and deeper extensions of the tumor in the prevertebral plane.
2. **CT and MR angiography** has mostly replaced conventional CT or MR for vascular tumors. In CT angio, the study is generally done in three phases—arterial, venous, and delayed. The delayed phase is comparable to a regular contrast enhanced CT and gives an idea of the soft tissue extensions of the tumor. A higher dose of contrast is used compared to regular CECT and thin slices (0.2 mm) are taken.
3. **(DSA) Digital subtraction angiography** (Invasive Angiography) has mostly been replaced by CT/MR angiography and is only reserved for those cases that may require balloon test occlusion (BTO) as a preparation for possible carotid artery resection, for embolization of highly vascular tumors and control of hemorrhage.

Carotid Body Tumor

1. Typically seen as a hypervascular lesion located at the bifurcation between ICA and ECA causing splaying of the two vessels (*Lyre sign*)—best appreciated in

© The Author(s) 2018
U. Nayak et al., *Clinical Radiology of Head and Neck Tumors*,
https://doi.org/10.1007/978-981-10-5036-7_11

arterial phase of CT angiography. In familial types, they may be bilateral and may also be associated with other paragangliomas. In syndromic paragangliomas, further imaging must be done to rule out pheochromocytoma.

2. Tumors are staged according to the Shamblin type of classification (type I, II, III) based on CT findings.
3. On T2 MR, they have a salt and pepper appearance (Salt: high signal foci of slow flow or hemorrhage; Pepper: low signal flow voids).

Glomus Tumor

CT (venous phase) is more useful in evaluation of glomus tumors as these tumors are closely associated with bony canals and the base of skull.

1. Glomus jugulare—loss of crest of bone between carotid canal and jugular bulb (*Phelps Sign*) and widening of jugular foramen
2. Glomus tympanicum—CT temporal bone shows a rounded vascular mass on the cochlear promontory

Other Paragangliomas

Glomus intravagale tumors arise from the X nerve and are therefore located lateral to the carotid and generally push the vessel anteriorly.

Lymphovascular Malformations

MR is the preferred choice of imaging in lymphovascular malformation to differentiate between lymphangioma, hemangioma, and A-V malformation.

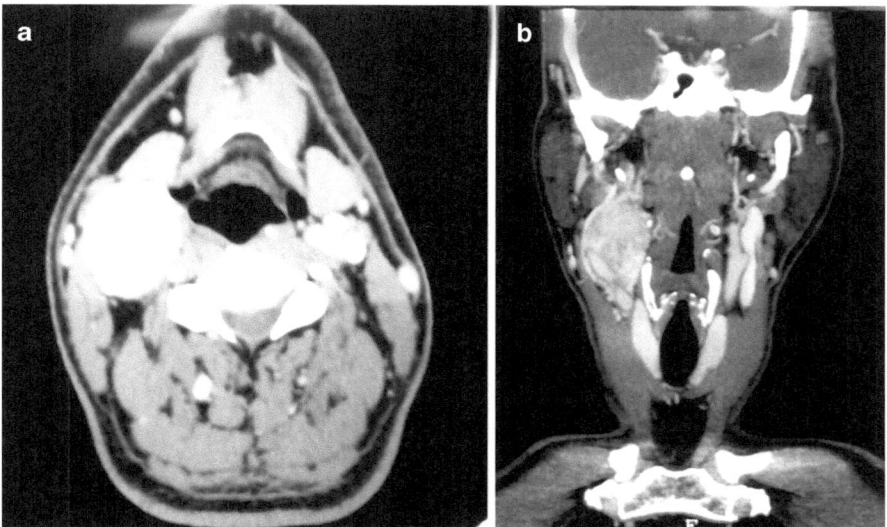

Fig. 11.1 (**a**) Carotid body tumor axial CT angio (arterial phase). (**b**) Carotid body tumor coronal reconstruction of same patient showing the longitudinal extent of the tumor

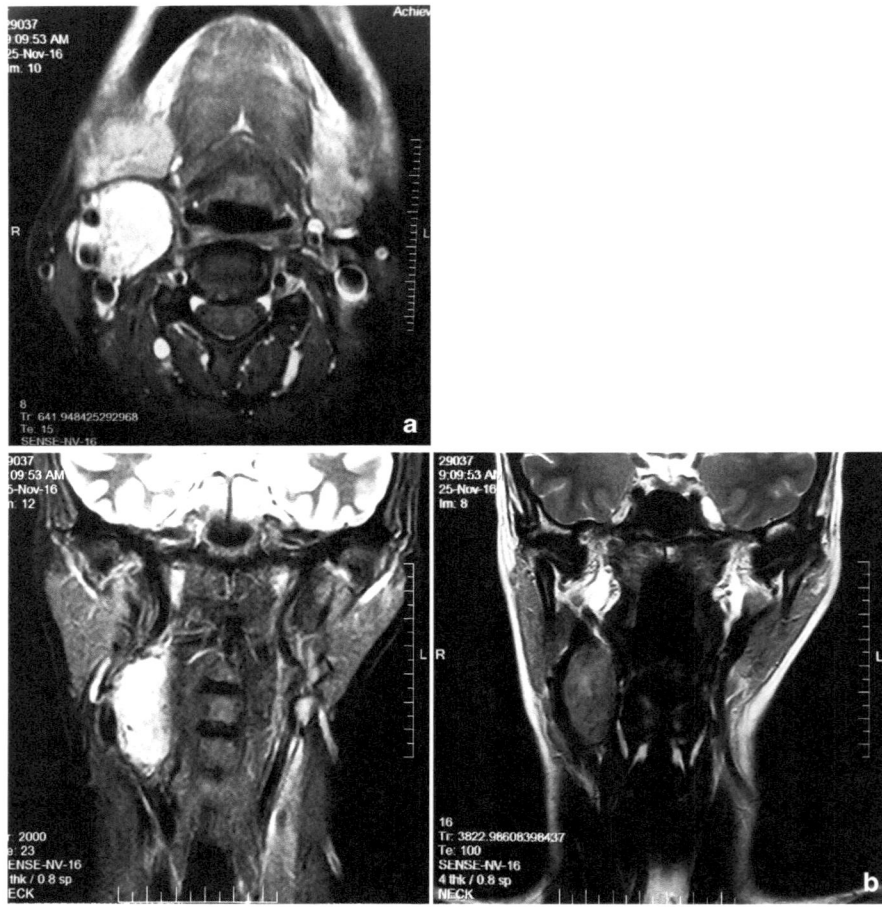

Fig. 11.2 (**a**) Carotid body tumor Axial T1 MR with contrast and fat suppressed showing typical location of tumor. (**b**) Same patient Coronal MR T1 contrast (*left*) and without contrast (*right*)

Fig. 11.3 Carotid body
tumor digital substraction
angiogram (DSA)
demonstrating tumor blush

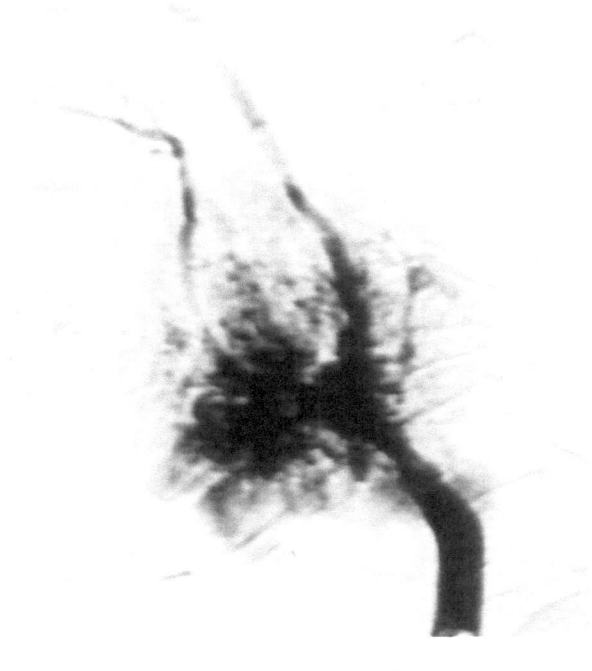

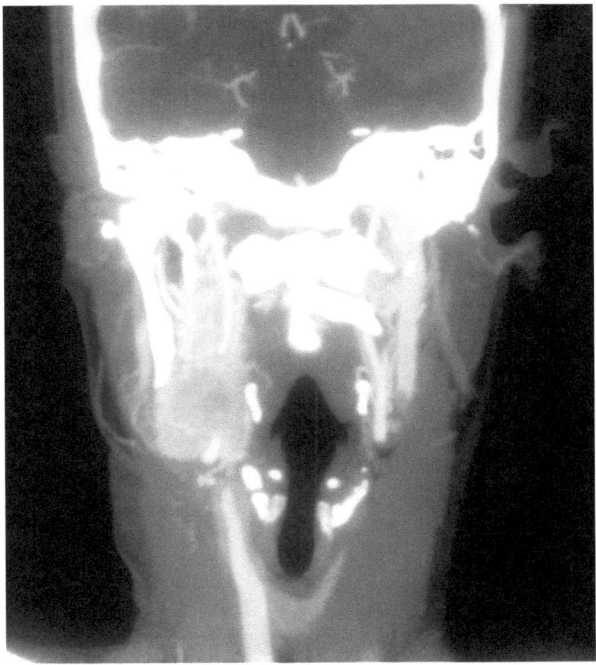

Fig. 11.4 Bilateral carotid
body tumor coronal CT
angio (venous phase)

Fig. 11.5 Bilateral carotid
body tumors CT angio
(delayed phase)

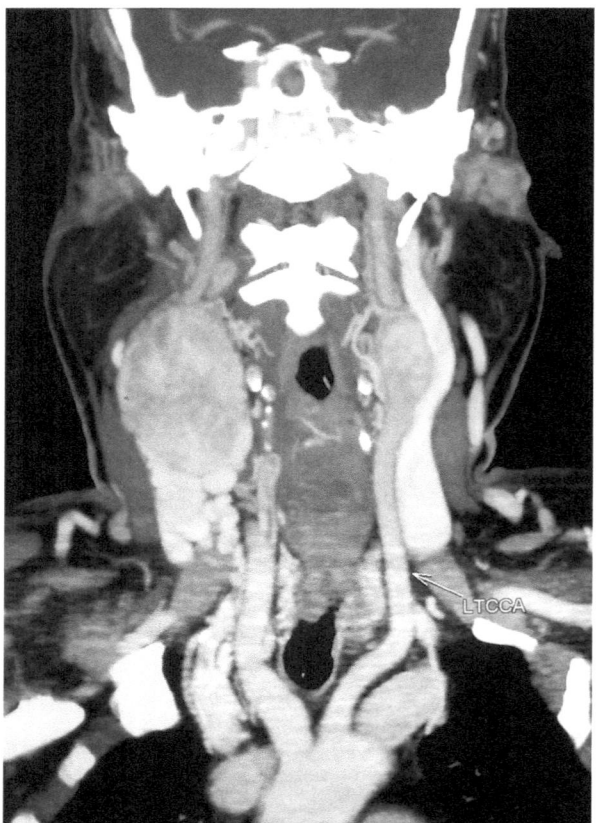

Fig. 11.6 Malignant carotid body tumor Axial CT - note complete (360 degree) encirclement of carotid artery (*red circle*) and prevertebral muscle involvement

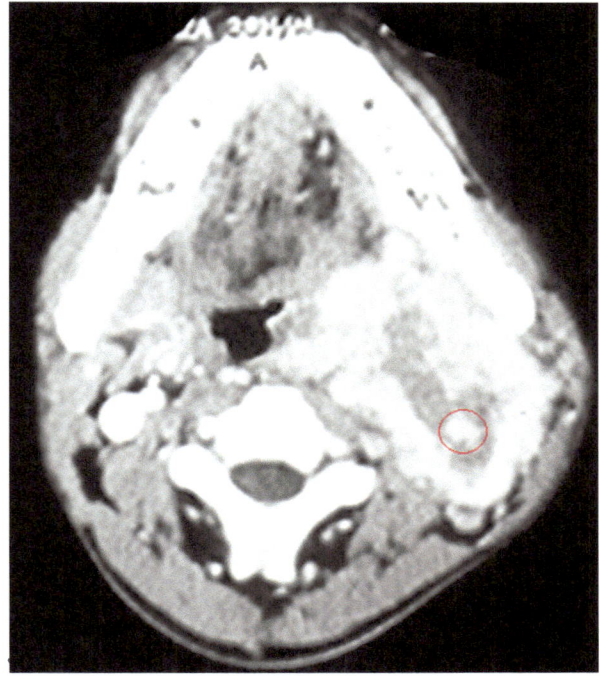

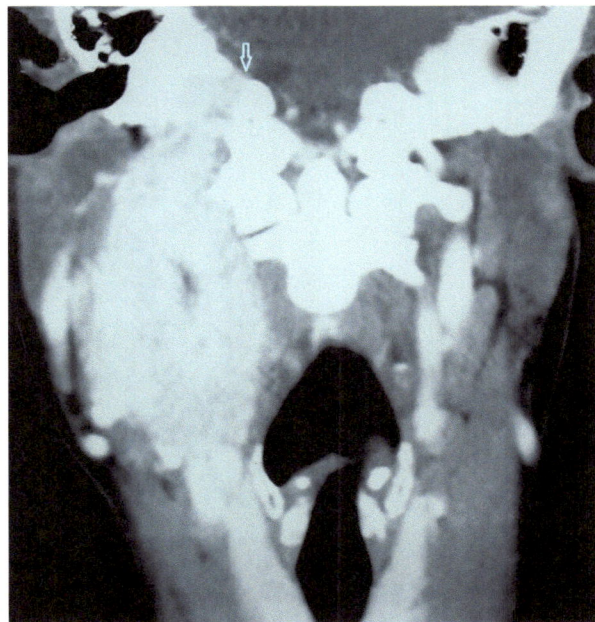

Fig. 11.7 Glomus tumor coronal CT angio (venous phase) showing large Glomus jugulare with widening of jugular foramen

Fig. 11.8 (**a**) Bilateral glomus tumors CT axial demonstrating widening of jugular foramen on *left side*. (**b**) Same patient coronal reconstruction

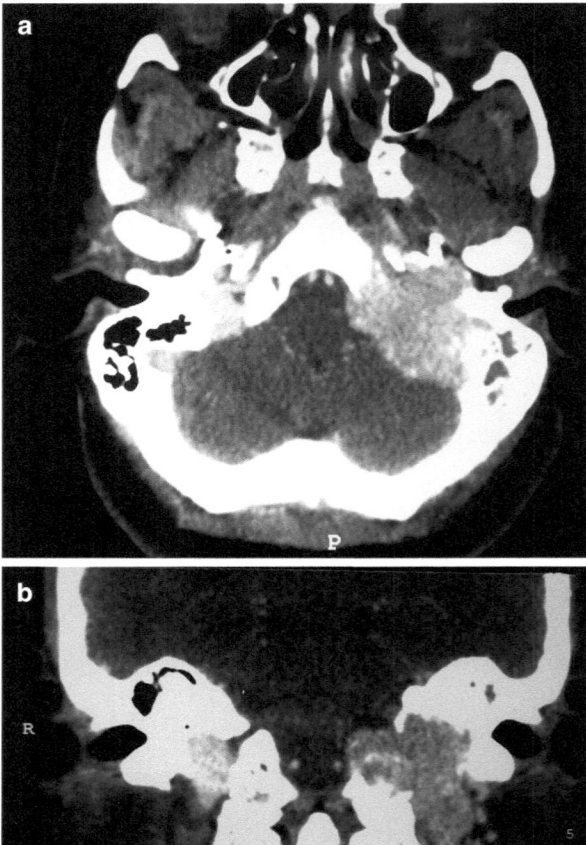

Fig. 11.9 Glomus intravagale coronal CT angio showing vagal paraganglioma. Note that the epicenter of the tumor is lateral to carotid artery

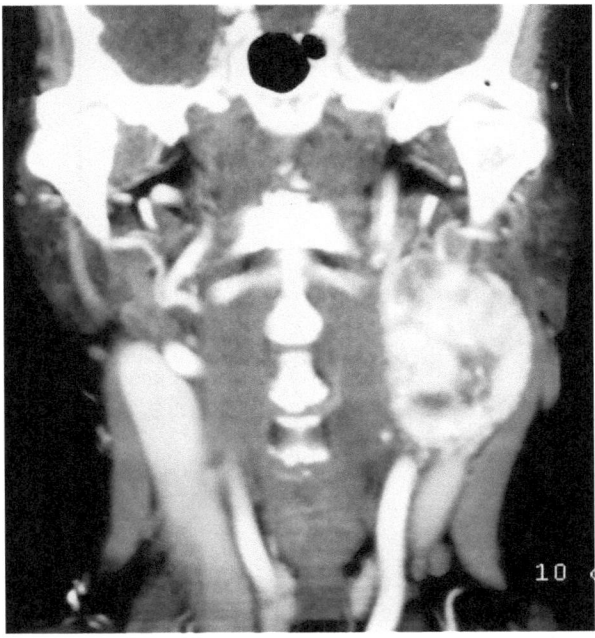

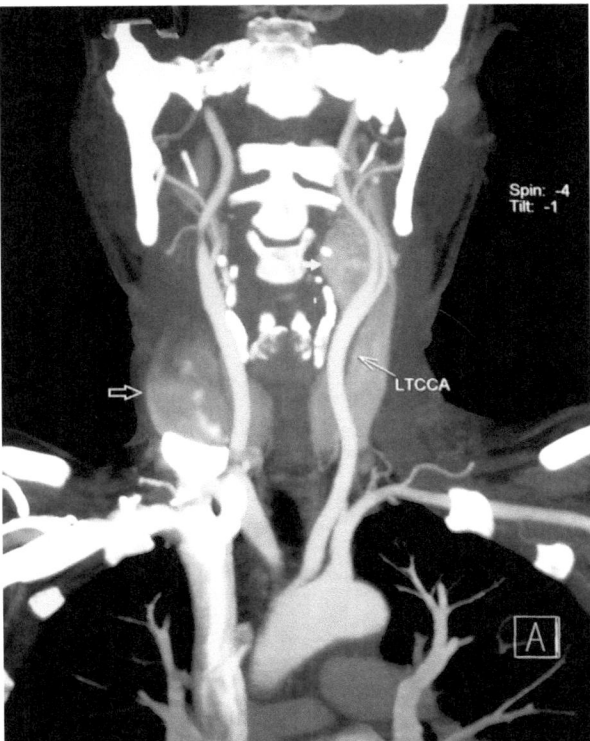

Fig. 11.10 CT angio (arterial phase) *right* paraganglioma and left carotid body tumor

Further Reading

1. Hanna E, Vural E, Prokopakis E, Carrau R, Snyderman C, Weissman J. The sensitivity and specificity of high-resolution imaging in evaluating perineural spread of adenoid cystic carcinoma to the skull base. Arch Otolaryngol Head Neck Surg. 2007;133(6):541–5.
2. Rumboldt Z, Gordon L, Gordon L, Bonsall R, Ackermann S. Imaging in head and neck cancer. Curr Treat Options Oncol. 2006;7(1):23–34.
3. Declercq A, Van den Hauwe L, Van Marck E, Van de Heyning PH, Spanoghe M, De Schepper AM. Patterns of framework invasion in patients with laryngeal cancer: correlation of in vitro magnetic resonance imaging and pathological findings. Acta Otolaryngol. 1998;118(6):892–5.
4. Beitler JJ, Muller S, Grist WJ, Corey A, Klein AM, Johns MM, Perkins CL, Davis LW, Udayasanker U, Landry JC, Shin DM, Hudgins PA. Prognostic accuracy of computed tomography findings for patients with laryngeal cancer undergoing laryngectomy. J Clin Oncol. 2010;28(14):2318–22.
5. Castelijns JA, Becker M, Hermans R. Impact of cartilage invasion on treatment and prognosis of laryngeal cancer. Eur Radiol. 1996;6(2):156–69.
6. Greess H, Lell M, Römer W, Bautz W. Indications and diagnostic sensitivity of CT and MRI in the otorhinolaryngology field. HNO. 2002;50(7):611–25.
7. Zbären P, Becker M, Läng H. Pretherapeutic staging of hypopharyngeal carcinoma. Clinical findings, computed tomography, and magnetic resonance imaging compared with histopathologic evaluation. Arch Otolaryngol Head Neck Surg. 1997;123(9):908–13.
8. Bailet JW, Abemayor E, Jabour BA, Hawkins RA, Ho C, Ward PH. Positron emission tomography: a new, precise imaging modality for detection of primary head and neck tumors and assessment of cervical adenopathy. Laryngoscope. 1992;102(3):281–8.
9. Weissman JL, Akindele R. Current imaging techniques for head and neck tumors. Review Article | Head & Neck Cancer| 01 May 1999.
10. Arya S, Chaukar D, Pai P. Imaging in oral cancers. Indian Journal of Radiology and Imaging. 2012;22(3):195–208.
11. Patkar D, Yanamandala R, Lawande M. Imaging in head and neck cancers. AIJOC. 2010;2(1):15–23.
12. Van den Brekel MWM, Castelijns JA. What the clinician wants to know: surgical perspective and ultrasound for lymph node imaging of the neck. Cancer Imaging. 2005;5:S41–9.

Books

13. Fleckenstein P, Tranum Jensen J. Anatomy in diagnostic imaging. 2nd ed. Copenhagen, Denmark: Munksgaard; 2010.
14. Harnsnerger H, Chistian Davidson H, Wiggins RH III, Macdonald AJ, Hudgins PA, Glastonbury CM, Michel MA, Curé JK, Swartz J, Branstetter B IV. Diagnostic imaging, head and neck. 1st ed. AMIRSYS Publication.
15. Moeller TB, Reif E. Pocket atlas of sectional anatomy, computed tomography and magnetic resonance imaging. Volume I: Head and neck. 3rd ed. Thieme Publication.
16. Dunnebier EA. Imaging for otolaryngologists. Volume I: Head and neck. 3rd ed. Noida, India: Thieme Publication, Thieme Medical and Scientific Publishers Private Ltd; 2014.